SPACE AND LIFE

An Introduction to
Space Biology and Medicine

SPACE AND LIFE

An Introduction to
Space Biology and Medicine

Hubert Planel

Professor Emeritus
School of Medicine
University of Toulouse (France)

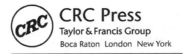

CRC Press
Taylor & Francis Group
Boca Raton London New York

CRC Press is an imprint of the
Taylor & Francis Group, an **informa** business

Originally published in French as *L'Espace et la Vie* by Hubert Planel.

CRC Press
Taylor & Francis Group
6000 Broken Sound Parkway NW, Suite 300
Boca Raton, FL 33487-2742

©Larousse, 1988.
© 2004 by Taylor & Francis Group, LLC
CRC Press is an imprint of Taylor & Francis Group, an Informa business

First issued in paperback 2019

No claim to original U.S. Government works

ISBN-13: 978-0-367-45437-1 (pbk)
ISBN-13: 978-0-415-31759-7 (hbk)

**Visit the Taylor & Francis Web site at
http://www.taylorandfrancis.com**

**and the CRC Press Web site at
http://www.crcpress.com**

Library of Congress Cataloging-in-Publication Data

Planel, Hubert.
    [Espace et la vie. English]
    Space and life / by Hubert Planel.
      p. cm.
    Includes bibliographical references and index.
    ISBN 0-415-31759-2 (alk. paper)
     1. Space biology. 2. Weightlessness. I. Title.

    QH327.P5213 2004
    571'.0919—dc22

                             2003065508

Library of Congress Card Number 2003065508

Foreword

When contemplating the amazing spectacle of a starry night one cannot help but ask the age-old question: *are humans and their fellow creatures the only living beings in the universe?* With the recent advent of space travel, it is now conceivable that humans might one day inhabit other planets or wander distant galaxies, exposed to environments previously unimagined. But can Earth's creatures live outside the protective atmosphere of our planet? How would they adapt to space? Could extraterrestrial life indeed exist? An attempt, albeit modest, will be made to answer these questions.

The space age was inaugurated over 40 years ago when the Soviet Union launched Sputnik-1 into orbit. Since then, both the Soviet Union and the United States have accomplished many historical "firsts." The Soviet Union launched the first artificial satellite and sent the first man into space, and a Soviet cosmonaut performed the first space walk. The American contribution includes the first man on the moon, the first reusable space vehicle, the space-based telescope and an impressive array of satellites for exploring the solar system. One of these, the COBE[1] satellite, has led to extraordinary revelations about the origin of the universe. The list is long and it soon becomes obvious, when comparing the merits of each country's tally, that there is no true "winner." However, it is not so much the past that deserves our focus. Rather, attention should be turned toward a future certain to be filled with extraordinary developments in space exploration.

One of the important questions to be addressed in this book is whether or not this future should lie only with unmanned exploration. Is human presence in space necessary? In astronomy, astrophysics, Earth observation, or telecommunications, the use of automated vehicles is often more efficient and appropriate. However, manned space flights have played and will continue to play an important role in the human conquest and use of space. They gave birth to the field of space medicine, which aims at ensuring human survival outside the Earth's atmosphere and gravitational field. In addition, space has emerged as a unique laboratory offering biologists and physiologists previously unimaginable research perspectives. In doing so, it has exposed living beings to a new set of environmental influences, including weightlessness. Thanks to space research, gravity is now recognized as a major factor of the terrestrial environment, the influence of which is felt throughout the biosphere. Enough research has been done to acquire fundamental knowledge about the effects of space flights. New scientific fields, such as gravitational biology and physiology, have made remarkable breakthroughs, and it is now possible to take stock of these results and observations.

---

[1] COBE: NASA's Cosmic Background Satellite measured temperature fluctuations or "bumps" in space, which are remnants of the big bang.

The aim of *Space and Life: An Introduction to Space Biology and Medicine* is to provide an overview of the main problems in space biology and medicine and to highlight some of the most striking data accumulated over the 40 years of research in this field. Of course quite a number of experimental results will go unreported, and the author asks any specialists shocked by these omissions to forgive him. Finally, in order to make space research results easier to understand, brief summaries of basic physiology and biology are given to help readers who are not well acquainted with these disciplines.

Acknowledgments

In setting up the first laboratory dedicated to space radiobiology and biology in France, I have over the years been in constant contact with European and American physicians and scientists. Thanks to them, I was able to gather the medical, biological and physical knowledge to write this book.

I thank the CNES (Centre National d'Études Spatiales), NASA, the Institute of Biomedical Problems in Moscow and the European Space Agency for their scientific and financial support.

I would like to express all my gratitude to Prof. Alexandre, G. Clément, A. Cogoli, C. Gharib, H. J. Marthy, G. Perbal and R. J. White for giving me a great deal of information on space biology and medicine.

I gratefully acknowledge my colleagues, Prof. J. P. Soleilhavoup, R. Tixador, G. Richolley, G. Gasset, F. Croute, Y. Blanquet and B. Pianezzi, who participated in space experiments carried out in my laboratory.

Finally, it has been a pleasure to work on this book with Gerardo Bautista and his staff. Last but not least, my thanks to Marie-Claire Prioleau, Zaia Mekki and Nelly Pons for typing the manuscript.

Hubert Planel

Contents

Chapter 1   Manned and Unmanned Missions 1

The Importance of Space and Astronautics 1
Human Presence in Space 2
Tribute to Space Shuttle Columbia 5

Chapter 2   Manned Space Flights.. 7

The First Men in Space 7
"One Giant Leap for Mankind" 9
Soviet Hopes 10
The First Accidents 12
Apollo-13 13
Challenger 14
The Future.. 17

Chapter 3   Space: An Extreme Environment... 21

The First Minutes of a Space Flight 21
The Space Environment and Flight-Related Factors 23
Reentry.. 24
Space Biology and Medicine 25

Chapter 4   Gravity and Weightlessness 27

Galileo and Newton.. 27
Free-Fall and Space Flights.. 28
Konstantin Tsiolkovsky and Jules Verne.. 31
Simulating and Creating Weightlessness on Earth 33
Simulating Microgravity... 34

Chapter 5   Physiological and Biological Effects of Weightlessness
in Humans and Animals. The Cardiovascular System 37

The First American Tests... 37
The First Soviet Tests 39
Basic Concepts in Physiology 39
The Effects of Gravity... 41
The First Effects of Weightlessness 43
Time Course of Cardiovascular Responses... 45

Chapter 6 The Skeletal System and Weightlessness 49

Bone Development and Restructuring 49
The Role of Hormones 53
The Influence of Gravity 54
The Effects of Space Flights 55
Animal Experiments 57
A New Model 59
Risks and Countermeasures...60
Conclusion 61

Chapter 7 The Muscular System 63

Muscle Fibers 63
Muscle Contraction..64
The Effects of Gravity 64
The Effects of Weightlessness...65
Conclusion 68

Chapter 8 The Vestibular Apparatus and Balance System...........................69

Proprioception..69
The Vestibular System 70
The Effects of Weightlessness...74
Adaptation and Plasticity of Nerve Centers..77
The Importance of Cognitive Phenomena 78
A Short Course in Comparative Anatomy and Physiology..................................80

Chapter 9 The Other Effects of Weightlessness..83

Blood and Weightlessness 83
The Effects of Space Flights 84
The Immune Response and Weightlessness...87
The Effects of Space Flights 88
Respiration and Weightlessness...90
Other Manifestations 91
Conclusion 92
Spin-Offs for Standard Medicine 95

Chapter 10 Space Cell Biology 97

The Theoretical Arguments 97
The Results of Space Experiments 99
    Cell Division 99
    The Cell Membrane and Exchanges
    with the Extracellular Environment...101

The Cytoskeleton 102
Energy Metabolism 103
Genes 103

Chapter 11 The Effects of Gravity and Weightlessness on Plants 105

The Gravitropic Response 105
Effects of Weightlessness 108

Chapter 12 Developmental Biology 113

Amphibian Eggs 113
Sea Urchin and Fish Eggs 116
Mammals 117
Evolution and Gravity 117

Chapter 13 Cosmic Radiation 121

A Few Concepts in Physics 121
    The Discovery of Cosmic Radiation 121
    Composition of Cosmic Radiation 121
        Solar Wind 122
        Galactic Cosmic Rays 122
        Radiation Belts 123
    Primary and Secondary Cosmic Radiation 124
Radiation Biology: General Concepts 125
    The Effects of Ionizing Radiation 125
    Doses in Radiation Biology and Their Meaning 127
The Dosimetry of Cosmic Radiation 128
The Effects of Cosmic Radiation 131
Problems Related to Cosmic Radiation 132
    Solar Flares 132
    Heavy Cosmic Ions 133
    The Combined Effect of Cosmic Radiation and Weightlessness 137
    Delayed or Late Effects 138
Conclusion 140

Chapter 14 Extraterrestrial Life 141

Life in the Solar System 141
Mars 141
    Titan: A Model of Prebiotic Synthesis on Earth? 146
    Beyond Mars and Titan 148
    Meteorites and Comets 149
    Life Outside the Solar System 152
    Molecules in Space 154

The Search for Extraterrestrial Life and Habitable Planets 156
The Search for Intelligent Extraterrestrial Civilizations 157

Conclusion 161

Epilogue 163

References 165

Index 167

1 Manned and Unmanned Missions

Human presence has added a new dimension to the conquest of space but because manned flights are very costly, the question has been raised as to whether this presence is indispensable. Numerous examples suggest that it is.

THE IMPORTANCE OF SPACE AND ASTRONAUTICS

On October 4, 1957, the first man-made object, Sputnik-1, was launched into space. This Soviet satellite made an orbital flight at an altitude varying between 228 and 947 km and repeatedly emitted a beeping sound that was heard around the world. This essential date in the history of humanity heralded the birth of space exploration or "astronautics," which has since led to unimagined technological, scientific and even political upheavals.

The technological and scientific developments in astronautics have also had a significant economic impact. The Apollo program alone mobilized more than 200,000 workers for several years. In Europe, several thousand people work directly or indirectly for the ESA, the European Space Agency. France employs 1,200 people at the space center in Toulouse. Having become host to numerous space-related industries, Toulouse is now known as the "space capital" of France.

Another spin-off of the space program is satellite technology. Spy satellites can identify large nuclear missile silos or objects merely tens of centimeters in size. Remote sensing satellites can survey vast areas in a single sweep or detect coastal pollution on a planetary scale.

Satellites have also brought changes that have revolutionized daily life. Placed in a geostationary orbit of 36,000 km, satellites transmit portable cellular phone conversations between people on the same street, in the same city or on different continents. Only a few decades ago, submerged oceanic cables were the only means of telephone communication. Although cables last longer, they cannot always be used to reach remote areas. Automobiles are now equipped with GPS or global positioning system units that assist drivers in their navigation. Satellite maps are routinely used for precise meteorological forecasts on television, a medium that has also dramatically changed in the space era. Programs increasingly transcend conventional cultural borders to bring viewers new information and perspectives.

Satellites are also valuable tools for scientists. Explorer-1, the first American satellite launched on January 31, 1958, may have seemed small—weighing only 8 kg compared to the 83 kg of Sputnik-1—yet it led to the important discovery of the Van Allen belts, the delineated zones of radiation around the Earth. Beyond techniques such as adaptive optics, which reduce distortion and improve observation from Earth, astronautics has become inseparable from astronomical research. The crowning example of this is the Hubble space telescope, which has recently led to a better understanding of stars and galaxies.

Based on the contributions of engineers and scientists working tirelessly in their ground-based offices and laboratories, it might be tempting to sum up astronautics as nothing more than a magnificent technical achievement or just another manifestation of Homo sapiens' intelligence. This is only partly true. Indeed, when Gagarin and the astronauts of the early period inaugurated the era of manned flights, the technical feat also became a new human adventure. From then on, the men and women who actively participated in the development of astronautics risked their lives, adding a new dimension to the conquest of space. The information received from the Voyager probes or the images of Halley's comet transmitted by the Giotto probe are certainly amazing, but nothing can compare with the emotion shared by millions of people on July 21, 1969 when Neil Armstrong stepped on the surface of the moon.

Despite the clear human contribution to space exploration, debate over the usefulness of manned missions continues. Economically, space missions are expensive: launching the Ariane rocket cost $150 million; the price of a major planetary mission is approximately $800 million; the cost of a shuttle flight is nearly $1 billion. Famous scientists such as Van Allen, after whom the radiation belts were named, have questioned the human presence in space, suggesting that more sophisticated robots should be sent into space instead. Since the flight of Sputnik-1, unmanned, automated spacecraft have routinely gathered and transmitted a lot of data back to Earth. Similarly, unmanned flights to distant planets such as Jupiter, Saturn or Uranus have been a source of remarkable scientific results. Owing to the duration of these flights and the fact that the crafts were not designed to return to Earth, the presence of astronauts onboard was unthinkable. Human presence can even interfere with certain types of missions. Instruments used for astronomical observations often require constant minute adjustments, and an astronaut simply moving about or sneezing could create accelerations that disturb the microgravity level within the spacecraft. Furthermore, near-weightless conditions are sometimes required to process certain pure state materials or to induce protein crystallization. In addition, as everyone knows, unmanned satellites are used for telecommunication and remote sensing. The problem, however, is not so simple. While unmanned and manned missions often serve their own particular purpose, they may also at times complement one another.

HUMAN PRESENCE IN SPACE

Man's conquest of space can be seen to some extent as a philosophical challenge. Human beings have always distinguished themselves from other living creatures by an insatiable thirst for knowledge and exploration. The first men who roamed the valleys of East Africa a million years ago left their birthplace to conquer the planet little by little, driven by a curiosity and yearning for richer territories and more temperate climes. Space can be considered to be an essential stage of this great adventure.

There are also technological justifications for human presence in space. A robot entirely capable of replacing man's versatility in space research does not yet exist. Grasping a syringe, injecting its contents into a cellular culture and then placing the culture into a refrigerated container is a task that could easily be automated. But during the Challenger D1 mission, the astronaut who did exactly that for a human lymphocyte experiment carried out twelve other biological experiments. A single human being can perform a variety of tasks during a flight where several robots would have been required. Would it have been less costly to automate so many functions?

Even with the recent progress in robotics, automated machines can only function within the constraints of a well-defined program. They are closed systems. On the other hand, humans are open to the outside world, they are capable of understanding their environment and reacting to unforeseen situations, as did the astronauts aboard Apollo-13. If the operations performed during a space flight are controlled from the ground, the transmission time depends on the distance between the spacecraft and the Earth. An order originating from a command center will reach Mars in 20 minutes, and the response will return to Earth in the same amount of time. These 40 minutes can be without consequence during a trouble-free automated mission. But if an accident or an unforeseen event were to require an immediate solution, the success of the mission might well be jeopardized. In the much more frequent case of orbital flights, the value of human presence becomes obvious when there are equipment failures, as a few well-known examples illustrate.

This type of malfunction occurred when NASA launched Skylab-2 into space on May 13, 1973. Only tens of seconds after lift-off, the micrometeoroid shield designed to protect the craft from interplanetary dust particles broke off, taking with it one of the solar array wings and damaging the second. When crew members Charles Conrad, Joseph Kerwin and Edward White rendezvoused with Skylab-11 days later aboard an Apollo capsule, they were faced with a difficult challenge. The temperature inside Skylab was 50°C and the damaged solar array wing had not been properly deployed, with the result that electricity production was seriously reduced. After surveying the damage, the astronauts first sought to protect the surface of Skylab from solar rays. During an EVA, extra-vehicular activity or space walk, the astronauts were able to surround the station with an aluminium-lined nylon sheet to lower the temperature inside the craft. During another EVA, the astronauts deployed the remaining solar array wing, reestablishing the electrical current necessary for the operation of the equipment onboard. Skylab had been salvaged.

The Salyut-7 orbital space station is another example of the necessity for human problem solving ability. Shortly after the crew, Kieim, Soloviev and Atkov, returned to Earth in 1984, a failure in the entire electrical circuit system occurred aboard the station. When the replacement crew, Dzhanibekov and Savitskaya, arrived in June of that year, they discovered a station at sub-zero temperature without light or ventilation. Following ground control instructions, the cosmonauts proceeded to modify the electrical circuits and reestablished the connections between the solar array wing and the batteries of the space station. Power was restored and the lights slowly came back on. Salyut-7, after having been considered lost, was once again operational. It is very unlikely that a robot could have made such repairs.

The spectacular repairs on the American Solar Max satellite and, more recently, the Hubble space telescope, provide yet further examples of the undeniable place of human presence in space. Solar Max—short for Solar Maximum Satellite—was launched on February 14, 1980. It was an exceptional machine, equipped with very precise instruments: a gamma spectrometer, an X-ray spectrometer and a UV spectrometer for studying the sun's corona during a period of maximum solar activity. Merely six months after its launch, Solar Max had revolutionized knowledge in solar physics, leading to the discovery of extraordinary magnetic disturbances capable of disrupting the solar atmosphere. These disturbances are analogous to the cyclones and anticyclones, which result from changes in atmospheric pressure and affect the Earth's climate. Solar Max had also gathered precious information about the temperature of the sun. Data from these experiments were still being collected when a mundane short circuit occurred in the electrical system. It was feared that the $75 million probe would just be lost in space, not to mention the cost of replacement. As an alternative, the possibility of recovery and repair was raised.

With some foresight, Solar Max had been equipped with a tethering device that would allow the satellite to be captured, brought back to Earth for repair and then relaunched. However, NASA decided on a different course of action: they would attempt to repair Solar Max in space. On April 10, 1984, the Challenger shuttle maneuvered to within 80 m of Solar Max. During a first EVA, G. Nelson and S. Van Hoften tried unsuccessfully to attach a metal anchor to the tethering device. Nelson next attempted to immobilize it by spraying it with several bursts of liquid nitrogen from bottles attached to his floating chair. This also failed and Solar Max began spinning uncontrollably, forcing the astronauts to abandon their attempt. They realized that Solar Max must first be brought under control with the robotic arm of the shuttle. Two days later, T. Hart exited the craft and finally succeeded in hauling the satellite into the shuttle bay. Later, Van Hoften and Nelson removed a protective plate and several screws, cut some wires and discovered that the piece designed for tethering Solar Max was 3 cm shorter than expected, explaining their earlier difficulty. On April 12, repairs were completed and Solar Max was redeployed in space. It was a major triumph. Repairing Solar Max was undeniably a great accomplishment, providing further evidence for the importance of man in space.

Several years later, astronauts were sent on a similar mission to carry out the highly publicized repair of the Hubble space telescope. The latter was launched in April 1990 and placed in orbit at an altitude of 570 km. Because it was orbiting beyond the Earth's atmosphere, the 13-m telescope was expected to provide observations unobtainable on the ground. Unfortunately, it was quickly discovered that the images transmitted by the telescope were out of focus due to a problem with its central mirror. It was feared that Hubble, as well as the dreams it fostered, would have to be abandoned.

Once again, NASA decided to attempt a repair operation in space. On December 2, 1993, a team of seven astronauts under the command of Richard Covey flew aboard the Endeavor shuttle and rendezvoused with Hubble. Two days later, the Swiss astronaut, Claude Nicollier, used the robotic arm to seize and immobilize the telescope. Jeff Hoffman and 59-year-old space veteran Story Musgrave changed four large gyroscopes during the first EVA. In another EVA, Kathy Thornton removed a damaged solar array wing and released it into space. "It looks like a bird," she said of the object that was seven times larger than herself. Thanks to a total of five EVAs and the crew's great skill, the telescope was not only completely repaired but also upgraded with new cameras and increased memory capacity in its central computer. The results were remarkable. The Hubble space telescope is now sending clear images. For example, it transmitted images of the collision of the Shoemaker-Levy comet with Jupiter, which led to extraordinary astronomical findings.

Since Hubble was repaired in 1993, three other missions have taken place with the help of the shuttle: one in February 1997, another in December 1999 and a more recent mission in February 2002. There again, extravehicular outings were necessary, not only to provide new equipment such as a space telescope imaging spectrograph, a near-infrared camera and a more powerful computer, but also to repair or replace defective equipment. Thus the gyroscopes, which are essential for the positioning of Hubble, were replaced during the third mission. Man will remain indispensable for future maintenance missions until a second-generation space telescope is launched. It is clear that missions that were originally planned simply for maintenance have become over the years repair missions. Without this type of manned mission, the space telescope would have ceased being operational a long time ago. The satellite LDEF (long duration exposure flight) provides yet another example. Without man's intervention, it could not have been brought back by the American shuttle after 69 months in space. By the way, it is worth noting that the Artemia shrimp embryos placed onboard in the form of cysts were later able to develop successfully on Earth!

Thanks to their numerous EVAs, astronauts also play an essential role in the construction of the International Space Station (ISS). By welcoming men and women from many different countries, the ISS represents the largest space program based on wide-scale international cooperation. Because it is important that a climate of trust exist between the various participating nations, the ISS project is obviously important from a political point of view.

In summary, many results presented here show that astronauts, in performing tasks that require intelligence, play an indispensable role in space. Yet there is another reason to support the presence of men and women aboard a spacecraft: they give us the possibility of increasing our knowledge in physiology and medicine. Space has become a laboratory for studying the response of living organisms to weightlessness and, as such, provides scientists and doctors with a unique and irreplaceable study tool. Space environment can be simulated to a certain extent on the ground but only during space flights can weightlessness truly be experienced.

TRIBUTE TO SPACE SHUTTLE COLUMBIA

After this book was written a new tragic accident occurred in the sky of the United States. On February 1, 2003, the space shuttle Columbia broke up, 15 minutes before its scheduled landing at Kennedy Space Center in Florida. Seven astronauts perished: Commander Rick D. Husband; Pilot William C. McCool; Payload Commander Michael P. Anderson; Mission Specialists David M. Brown, Kalpana Chawla, and Laurel Clark; and Israel's first astronaut, Payload Specialist Ilan Ramon.

Columbia was the oldest of NASA shuttles, first launched in 1981. It was on its 28th mission. It underwent an extensive overhaul in 1998–1999.

The causes of the accident are still unknown, but temperature and pressure telemetry recording sensors indicated the start of an unusual temperature increase in the left main landing door and a loss of pressure on the left outboard and inboard tires. For some officials, the accident could be due to a piece of foam that came off during takeoff, striking the left wing of Columbia.

Just after Columbia broke up, debris fell down in East Texas. Debris was also found as far as Louisiana, Arkansas, Arizona, New Mexico, and California. The debris fell down in fields, houses, and even on a dentist performing surgery in Nacogdoches, Texas. Fortunately, noone was injured. By no later than March 27th, 42,000 pieces of debris had been found. Some of them weighed several tens of kilograms. Meanwhile, the search for debris continues.

After the Columbia accident, flights of American shuttles were temporarily stopped. Meanwhile, additional investigations are in progress. Astronauts will fly in the Russian Soyuz, and material will be carried by the spacecraft Progress. In this way, the International Space Station Program could go on as well as international cooperation in space research.

2 Manned Space Flights

Humans have always sought new continents and oceans to explore, and the conquest of space is a logical extension of this quest. Men and women have witnessed the most important moments in this new adventure, and these moments will be remembered not only in the history of space flights but in the history of mankind.

THE FIRST MEN IN SPACE

Space biology and medicine is more closely linked to progress in astronautics and manned flights than to any other field. This warrants a brief review of the important events in space exploration, which include both successes and failures.

The Soviet Union launched the first man into space but its manned space program did not get off to a promising start. Valentina Bondarenko burned to death in an oxygen-filled airtight chamber during a ground-based simulation experiment, and Piotr Dolgov was killed in a failed parachute jump. These tragic events left only two candidates for the first manned flight: Yuri Gagarin and Gherman Totov. Gagarin was selected on April 10, 1961.

In spite of these accidents, the success of Gagarin's flight was likely since it was already known that living creatures could withstand space and weightlessness. Laika (Figure 1), the dog who flew aboard Sputnik-2 on November 3, 1957, had survived

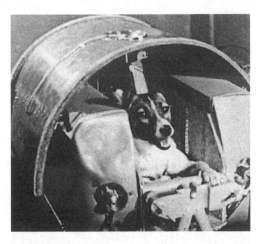

FIGURE 1 *Laika*
Laïka was the first mammal to fly in space. Laïka was launched aboard Sputnik-2 on November 3, 1957. (From Institute of Biomedical Problems, Moscow.)

7

the orbital flight. Several years later in August 1960, two other dogs, Strelka and Belka, accompanied by a few rats and mice, flew aboard the Korabl-2 rocket and were safely recovered after the ejection of the passenger module. Both dogs, Chernushka and Zvesdoshka, who flew, respectively, on March 9 and 21, 1961, returned to Earth in good health. There were, however, some disturbing mechanical failures. In May of the previous year, the fortunately unmanned Vostok-1 failed to return to Earth. On July 23, 1960, a launch failed and during the same year, Korabl-3 burned up during its reentry into the atmosphere, killing dogs Pchelka and Mushka. The same month, the third stage of a rocket failed to fire. However, Gagarin had complete confidence in Serguei Korolev, the engineer in charge of constructing the Vostok launchers. This man was to play an essential role in the history of Soviet space flights until his premature death in 1966.

Gagarin's inaugural flight, which lasted 1 hour 48 minutes, was a success (Figure 2). He circled the Earth one and a half times at a maximum altitude or apogee of 327 km and a minimum altitude or perigee of 175 km. There was only one problem during the entire flight. Shortly after he went into orbit, radio contact between Korolev and Gagarin was interrupted due to an error in transmission between two tracking stations. When Gagarin landed at 7:55 a.m. in the Saratov region, the first person he saw upon exiting his capsule was a peasant working in a field.

Gagarin was 27 years old when he flew into space and made history. He was an air force officer, as were many of the later Soviet cosmonauts. He was immediately hailed as a Soviet hero and was acclaimed in many other countries as well. On several occasions he said he wanted to fly again but on March 27, 1968, seven years after orbiting the Earth, Gagarin died piloting a MIG 15 on a training flight only a few hundred kilometers from Moscow.

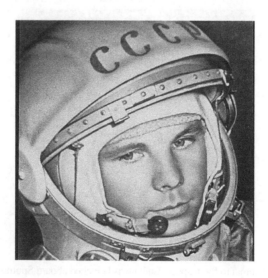

FIGURE 2 *Gagarin*

Yuri Alekseevitch Gagarin, the first man launched into space on an orbital mission. (From Institute of Biomedical Problems, Moscow.)

Another important date in the history of space flights is March 18, 1965 when Alexei Leonov floated freely in space outside his Voskhod-2 spacecraft. Leonov thus performed the first space walk. He exited through an airlock and, wearing a space suit equipped with a built-in oxygen tank, drifted 5 m from the craft. When the light from the sun unexpectedly blinded him he was soon drenched in sweat, and Leonov wanted to return to the craft. During his exit, however, his space suit had slowly expanded and Leonov could no longer fit through the airlock. He slowly depressurized his suit and, after several minutes of exhausting effort, was finally able to return inside Voskhod. The space walk lasted 12 minutes. Thanks to his courage and skill, Leonov had overcome great difficulties and accomplished an extraordinary technological and human feat.

"ONE GIANT LEAP FOR MANKIND"

After Gagarin and Leonov's flights, the Soviet Union had undeniably won the first two rounds in the conquest of space. John Kennedy, then President of the United States, understood that the next step in prestige was the conquest of the moon. President Kennedy wanted to overcome the feeling of humiliation the Soviet successes had brought on America. On May 25, 1961, with only Alan Shepherd's 15-minute sub-orbital flight to NASA's credit and against the advice of many experts, he declared:

"I believe that this nation should commit itself to achieving the goal, before the decade is out, of landing a man on the moon and returning him safely to Earth. No single space project in this period will be more impressive to mankind, or more important for the long-range exploration of space, and none will be so difficult or expensive to accomplish."

These words signalled the start of the Apollo program, which would mobilize more than 200,000 people and stimulate American industry. The Apollo manned flights began after seven years of relentless labor. The Apollo-7 mission in October 1968 and the Apollo-9 mission in March 1969 were both circumterrestrial flights. Apollo-8 and Apollo-10, on the other hand, flew around the moon in December 1968 and May 1969, respectively.

The most important step in astronautics since Leonov's flight was engraved in human history on July 16, 1969, only 8 years after Kennedy's speech. On that day, Neil Armstrong (Figure 3), an American civil aviation test pilot, and Edwin Aldrin, an air force colonel, landed the lunar module (LM) of the Apollo-11 mission on the surface of the moon at the Sea of Tranquillity. Pausing at the bottom of the ladder, Armstrong spoke words that were to be immortalized: "That's one small step for Man, one giant leap for Mankind." During the next two hours, Armstrong and Aldrin planted the American flag on the lunar surface, set up scientific equipment, took numerous photographs and collected 22 kg of lunar soil.

It was a remarkable success for the two men and for the United States, yet it was nearly overshadowed by another event. As Aldrin and Armstrong were preparing to return to Earth, extraordinary news was announced. The Jodrell Bank telescope in Great Britain had received signals transmitted from Luna-15, an unmanned Soviet probe making its way toward the moon. Luna-15 was equipped with an automated

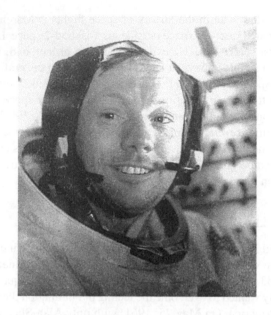

FIGURE 3 *Neil Armstrong*

Neil Armstrong, the first man to walk on the moon on July 21, 1969. (From Institute of Biomedical Problems, Moscow.)

cargo trunk designed to gather lunar samples and bring them back to Earth. It was due to return before the American astronauts, thereby lessening the importance of their accomplishment. However, the Soviet dream was short-lived. They had miscalculated the orbit of the spacecraft, and Luna-15 crashed on the surface of the moon, 800 km from the American landing site. The Soviet flight illustrates the extent of the competition between the two superpowers in the conquest of space.

The lunar landing and the majority of the Apollo program missions were successful. Six flights followed Apollo-11, 12 astronauts stayed on the moon for a total of 160 hours, traveling 95 km on foot or in the lunar rover. They brought back 380 kg of samples, took more than 30,000 photographs and deposited on the lunar surface enough equipment to perform about 60 scientific experiments. Yet the Apollo program was eventually cancelled and the last three planned flights never took place. At that time, the United States was preparing to launch Skylab and was discussing programs such as the Shuttle. Another policy—less ambitious and less costly—was being elaborated.

SOVIET HOPES

In the face of the success of American manned missions, the Soviet Union directed public attention to its successes with unmanned probes. This Soviet focus began to influence some American experts who did not support manned lunar missions. The success of the Apollo program did not defeat the Soviet Union. Indeed, the Soviets inaugurated unmanned probe missions to the moon. In September 1959, the Luna-2 probe studied the lunar magnetic field and cosmic radiation and then crashed on the moon. One month later, Luna-3 transmitted photographs of the moon's dark side. After the Luna-15 mission competing with Armstrong and Aldrin had failed, the Soviets successfully landed an automated vehicle on the lunar surface. This probe, the Lunakhod, was able to move across the moon's dusty surface and take samples. However, Lunakhod traveled 10 km in 10 months while the manned lunar rover had covered 3 km in only 3 days. This difference in efficiency provides more evidence for the superiority of manned over robotic missions, in those days at any rate.

Although Soviet authorities claimed that sending unmanned probes into space was a deliberate choice, it was later revealed that the USSR had indeed hoped to send manned missions to the moon, even though the Apollo program had a significant head start. The cosmonaut Vladimir Komarov, who had already flown in October 1964 aboard the first Voskhod, supposedly declared: "*I can confirm that the Soviet Union will not be defeated by the United States in the race to put a man on the moon... For the United States, the expected date is 1969 + x but ours is 1969 + x − 1.*"

During the 1950s and 1960s, the Russian space program was under the direction of Sergei Korolev. He was responsible for every Soviet success during that period. While the United States was involved in the Apollo program, Korolev, a remarkable engineer, designed a spacecraft for three astronauts. The craft comprised a command module, a service module and a one-man lunar landing module. A manned lunar mission was planned to coincide with the fiftieth anniversary of the Soviet Union in the second half of 1967. Unfortunately, Korolev died while the lunar craft was still under construction. His death had serious consequences. The test of a new and very powerful launcher failed, and it was only in September 1968 that the lunar flight could have taken place. This was an automated flight. The spacecraft, called Zond, was a modified version of the Soyuz ships used for manned flights. Zond landed on the Indian Ocean. In December 1969, a second flight took place, which was also unmanned. This time it was successful and landed in Soviet territory, as had all previous manned Soviet flights.

The Soviets abandoned their lunar program once they realized that they could not compete with the Americans. The latter's craft had long been able to maneuver easily in space, a capacity essential for landing on the moon and docking with the return module afterwards. In the beginning of the astronautics era, the Soviets concentrated their efforts on rocket development while the Americans, beginning with the Gemini flights, developed sophisticated craft equipped with very advanced electronics. By the beginning of the Apollo program, NASA already had a technological advance over its Soviet counterpart.

The intense competition between the United States and the Soviet Union may seem absurd today. However, the historical importance of the two nation's contributions to human expansion into space will not be forgotten. As both the cost and importance of space flight missions have increased, the two nations have learned to cooperate. Perhaps in a hundred years, the inhabitants of lunar or Martian space stations will have lost their terrestrial nationality and the nationalism that goes with it. Meanwhile, the ISS is the emblem of the cooperation that is being fostered between nations.

THE FIRST ACCIDENTS

Although the United States and the Soviet Union had many successes, both had their share of accidents. Overall, there have been very few disasters, but those that did occur were often dramatic. The Challenger incident, for example, was engraved in the memory of an entire generation. Unfortunately, it was not the only tragedy of this type.

After a series of successful Mercury (1961–1963) and Gemini flights (1965–1966), NASA launched the Apollo program. On January 21, 1967, Virgil ("Gus") Grissom, who had already flown in 1961 and 1965, Edward White, the first American to perform an EVA, and Roger Chaffee, a Corvette captain, took their seats in the Apollo-1 capsule on top of the Saturn rocket in the launch area. The gas tanks of the rocket were empty since this was simply a prelaunch test. For six hours the astronauts were strapped in their seats, wearing their space suits. Everything seemed to be working normally when Chaffee suddenly screamed "Fire! Fire!" into his microphone. Other words and cries for help were also probably spoken before the cabin went forever silent.

The fire is believed to have been caused by a short circuit in the wiring beneath Grissom's feet. In a matter of seconds, the nets holding the astronauts' equipment caught fire, as did the cabin lining, the seats and the electric cables in spite of the fact that they were all supposedly made of inflammable material. Since the atmosphere in the cabin was pure oxygen—this was typical of American space flights at the time—the fire spread rapidly. It is thought that the cabin burned in only 15 seconds. The autopsy showed that the astronauts died of asphyxiation.

Since this accident occurred on the ground, the question was raised as to whether or not the three astronauts could have been saved. It took approximately 15 minutes for rescuers to reach the cabin because the electrical current operating the tower elevators leading to the capsule had been cut. Several minutes went by before NASA personnel managed to open the exit hatch (for security reasons, this door could only be opened from the outside). Even if the rescuers had arrived immediately, they would have only found the burned bodies of the three men.

A replacement team was selected rapidly, even before the numerous improvements made to the Apollo capsules were completed. NASA thus responded to Grissom's fateful words, spoken after his Gemini-3 flight: *"We have a dangerous job, and we hope that if something happens to us that will not slow down the program. The conquest of space is worth risking your life over."* The Apollo-1 fire was the only accident on the ground; the others occurred in flight.

The first accident in space occurred during Vladimir Komarov's flight aboard Soyuz-1. The flight began normally, and the recordings during the first 12 hours showed that the cosmonaut tolerated the space environment very well. However, nearly half way through the flight, the spacecraft started rotating abnormally. Both ground control and Komarov attempted to correct the slowly increasing problem by modifying the orbit of the craft and delaying its reentry into the atmosphere. According to a technician working at an American military telecommunication base in Turkey, the cosmonaut was put in contact with his wife and the then Premier, Aleksei Kosygin. Reentry was then attempted. The cabin detached from the service module and began to fall, spinning like a top. The parachute did not open as its ropes had become tangled at an altitude of approximately 7 km, and the cabin crashed in a field in the Orenburg region. Overall, the flight lasted 26 hours and 17 minutes.

Four years later, the Soviet Union once again paid a heavy toll in its conquest of space when three Soviet cosmonauts died aboard Soyuz-11. Georgi Dobrovolsky, Vladislav Volkov and Victor Patsayev had been on the Salyut space station for 22 days when they began their return to Earth aboard the Soyuz craft, a shuttle docked to Salyut. The craft detached normally, but the valve that was due to equalize cabin pressure with atmospheric pressure at the end of the flight was inadvertently opened while the spacecraft was still in the vacuum of space. The air in the cabin escaped, causing the immediate death of the three cosmonauts by air embolism. When the news of this tragedy reached the community, the world's top scientists were gathered in Seattle for one of the most important international space conferences, the COSPAR.

It is difficult to imagine how a highly trained individual could make such a mistake, but an astronaut cannot execute all the tasks he is entrusted with always perfectly. Humans are prone to error, regardless of their level of training. For example, the astronauts who performed certain biological experiments in the Spacelab aboard the Challenger shuttle used the wrong syringe in an experiment with cells. During the same mission, they forgot to inseminate the culture medium for an experiment on bacterial resistance to antibiotics. These errors might have been the result of fatigue from the heavy workload as well as sleep deprivation. Weightlessness may also affect cerebral activity and alertness in unknown ways. There are no definite solutions to this problem, but such mistakes should certainly not discourage human involvement in the conquest of space.

APOLLO-13

The supposed bad luck associated with the number 13 certainly applied to the Apollo program. After the accident aboard Apollo-1, the Apollo missions that followed (both trial and lunar missions), were successful. However, the Apollo-13 mission was a fiasco although it luckily ended without human casualties.

Like its two predecessors, Apollo-13 was supposed to return to the moon. Apollo-13 was a complex piece of machinery, with a cylinder-shaped service module for storing fuel tanks, batteries, water, oxygen and most of the supplies. A cone-shaped command module above the service module provided enough space for the crewmembers, Jim Lovell, Jack Swingert and Fred Haise, to sit side by side. Further up, there was a lunar module (LM) at the tip of the command module. An airlock allowed the astronauts to move between the two compartments.

The problems began during the launch on April 11, 1970. Two minutes into the flight, the central engine of the Saturn rocket second stage suddenly stopped working. This meant the third-stage engine had to function longer than usual to compensate for the loss of power. This minor incident did not bring an end to the mission, and the craft continued its voyage to the moon. Shortly thereafter, the astronauts heard an explosion that set alarms ringing within the craft. "Houston, we've got a problem here," Lovell reported to ground base. A short circuit in the service module had set the isolating material of an oxygen tank on fire. The tank exploded and severely damaged the service module.

For the next two hours, the crew was without electricity or water. They finally sought refuge in the LM, which was larger than the command module and had its own batteries, water tanks and food. The LM was designed to land two astronauts on the moon and return them to the spacecraft. Once they had returned to the orbiting command and service modules, the LM would be jettisoned in space. During the crisis, the crewmembers were told to remain as long as possible in the LM. A major catastrophe had already been narrowly avoided.

At that point, the Apollo craft had begun to orbit the moon. On the ground, the entire NASA staff and members of the various companies that had participated in the craft's construction were working together to bring the astronauts safely back to Earth. As a first step, the flight plan was modified. Instead of landing on the moon, their priority was now to return to Earth. To accomplish this, the astronauts would use the lunar module engines to propel the entire Apollo craft toward Earth. On the sixth day, they separated from the service module and were able to take stock of the damage through the porthole. Several square meters of the outside of the module had been ripped and most of the inside had been destroyed. For the final Earth approach, the astronauts moved to the command module, since it was the only part of the craft with a heat shield capable of absorbing the heat generated during reentry. They closed the hatch and released the LM. The command module still had enough fuel to open the parachutes. As a result of this minute-by-minute problem solving, Lovell, Swigert and Haise were safely recovered in the Pacific Ocean after a disastrous six-day flight.

Using the LM as a rescue vehicle had saved the crew's lives. Apollo had also been equipped with another escape system, an accessory rocket fixed to the top of the command module. If there had been a problem with the Saturn rocket engine, the capsule could have separated from the rest of the Apollo craft. The accessory rocket could have then propelled it to an altitude high enough for the parachutes to be deployed. The space shuttles did not have such a launch escape system, the lack of which had tragic consequences.

CHALLENGER

One of the most dramatic accidents in space flight history occurred on January 28, 1986 when the Challenger space shuttle exploded suddenly, 73 seconds after its launch. Challenger's crew consisted of Commander Francis Scobee, pilot Michael Smith, the specialists Ellison Oniwuka, Ronald McNair, Gregory Jaris, and two women, Judith Resnik, who had flown on August 1984 aboard the Discovery shuttle, and Christa McAuliffe. Christa McAuliffe was a teacher who had been selected out of 11,000 candidates to report her experience in space to schoolchildren across America. The drama of the explosion was magnified by the fact that the accident occurred at low altitude. Family members and guests gathered at Cape Canaveral as well as the millions of television viewers who had tuned in to watch the first elementary school teacher fly into space witnessed the tragedy first hand. Many years have elapsed since the Shuttle's fateful 25th flight, and two questions asked at the time can now be answered. What happened? Could the accident have been avoided?

The Shuttle is propelled into orbit by a launcher consisting of three parts: an enormous tank filled with nearly 2 million liters of liquid hydrogen and two smaller booster rockets filled with propellant. Each booster has four compartments joined together by circular gaskets called O-rings. The Shuttle is mounted on the lower two thirds of the large tank, and the two boosters are fastened to the central tank on either side of the Shuttle. Most of the central tank and the boosters are situated behind the Shuttle nose, where the astronauts sit during the launch. The two boosters and the three main engines of the Shuttle are fed by the large central tank. A vast amount of energy is required to put its 100 tons into orbit. When the Shuttle is launched, the three engines and the booster engine ignite. The main engines generate 600 tons and each booster 1500 tons of thrust. The boosters work for two minutes before separating from the Shuttle and falling into the sea. They fall in the ocean off the Florida coast and are equipped with parachutes to slow their descent. The central tank is jettisoned at an altitude of 110 km and destroyed when it reenters the atmosphere. The Shuttle continues its trajectory into orbit using its two remaining engines.

On January 28, 1986, the Shuttle engines and boosters ignited six seconds sooner than the expected T-O s but the launch seemed to be a success and the Houston control center ordered: *"Challenger, full throttle."* Smith responded, *"Full throttle, Roger."* The trouble began soon after the launch.

Shortly after takeoff, a trail of white, then black smoke escaped from one of the booster lower-most O-rings. It disappeared after a couple of seconds. At $T+48$ s, the Shuttle encountered violent winds, stronger than those experienced on previous flights. The gusts lasted approximately 10 seconds. At $T+58$ s, the smoke reappeared in the same booster. One second later, the smoke gave way to flames. The vibrations caused by the gusts of winds had widened a fissure in one of the booster O-rings. John Young, chief of the American corps of astronauts, surmised that the vibrations had also ruptured a device that attached the booster to the central tank. These devices are always submitted to very strong dynamic stress due to the thrust of the two boosters. In the case of Challenger, the rupture occurred at the same level as the damaged O-ring. The Shuttle could not recover from these events which would rapidly lead to its tragic explosion.

At $T+60$ s, three sensors situated in the compression chamber of the right booster detected a fall in pressure. To correct the Shuttle trajectory, the computers onboard increased the thrust of the left booster. Challenger then began to zigzag, pulling to the right, then to the left. Also at $T+60$ s, the size of the flame increased to a length of 12 m. Challenger was now rattling more and more due to the imbalance caused by the differential thrust of its engines. The fire had now spread to the entire length of the ring, and a large red glow appeared between the Shuttle and the booster, which was losing its fuel. The pressure in the central tank was falling.

At $T+67$ s, the O-ring was completely destroyed and replaced by a circle of fire. The booster mounting device, situated at the same level as the O-ring and damaged by the gusts of wind and the high temperature (about 900°C) caused by the fire, broke off.

At T+72 s, the booster wall ruptured, causing the rear section to flip and separate from the forward section, which was still attached to the central tank. The right wing of the Shuttle broke and the central tank was punctured near its hydrogen-filled base. Oxygen soon began to escape.

At T+73 s, the size of the flames along the large tank increased, and the explosion occurred. The Shuttle was ejected from the central tank. It had lost its wings and main engines but, according to the photographs taken a second after the explosion, the cabin seemed to be intact.

The cabin fell 14.5 km for two and a half minutes before breaking to pieces on hitting the ocean. The search carried out by aircraft helped recover the two boosters, half of the large central tank and most of the cabin, including large pieces of the fuselage, wings and doors. While the Houston control center was announcing the Shuttle launch failure, the two boosters that had continued their course independently were destroyed by remote control for security reasons.

Did the crew realize what was happening? They may not have worried about the pressure changes in the different engines, but they certainly must have felt the sudden changes in direction caused by the thrust differential. They could not have been aware of the leak in the boosters since it occurred at the rear of the craft, well away from the cabin. No communication with Houston was established except for the brief "oh, oh" spoken by Copilot Smith when the explosion occurred.

In the weeks following the accident, a commission headed by the former American Secretary of State, William Rogers, was created to determine the causes of the Challenger accident. Unlike the Apollo spacecraft, shuttles do not have a rescue rocket in case the cabin separates prematurely from the launcher. It was this type of device that saved the lives of Vasily Lazarev and Oleg Makarov on April 5, 1975 when, faced with a launcher malfunction, the Soyuz command module was able to separate quickly from the rest of the craft. The cosmonauts were recovered 1600 km away, in shock from the 18 *g* acceleration but alive. In the case of the Shuttle, the only emergency action possible if the shuttle engines do not fire is to separate the shuttle from the boosters and the central tank. Having reached an altitude of 40,000 m, it is then supposed to make a descent and land on the ocean. However, the astronauts' chances of survival are slim since shuttles were never designed for recovery at sea. Even if releasing the boosters might have limited the extent of the accident, suddenly stopping the Challenger flight at low altitude would still have presented a considerable risk.

After the Challenger accident, shuttle flights were postponed until January 1990. Challenger was replaced in May 1991 by a new shuttle, the Endeavor. Although numerous modifications were made, the flights did not get off to a promising start. The tanks leaked hydrogen the first time they were filled, causing some delay in the reestablishment of launches. Since then, the number of shuttle flights has increased rapidly. Some flights have also lasted longer than the standard one week.

Because humans are present on the shuttle flights, specialists in different disciplines have been able to develop scientific programs aboard shuttle flights. Numerous experiments in biology and physiology are regularly performed, especially during Spacelab missions. Spacelab is an experimental facility developed by Germany and the European Space Agency and is used as an orbiting laboratory for particular life science missions.

Spacelab features Biorak, a module used for biological experiments. It can also house another module, Anthrorack, which facilitates human physiology experimentation in flight. Thanks to this module, more than 19 cardiovascular, pulmonary and endocrine experiments were performed during the German D2 Spacelab mission in April 1993.

The Neurolab missions, carried out in May 1999 by American, European and Japanese scientists, focused on basic research issues in neuroscience. Such international programs can be considered as a first step in long-range plans to be extended on the ISS.

THE FUTURE

For years to come, unmanned space flights will play a part in the exploration and conquest of space. However, humans will also have a fundamental role in the future of space exploration. Indeed, the United States, Russia, Japan, Canada and Europe have united to construct the ISS. The ISS is an orbiting laboratory where observations in fields such as astronomy and experiments on the effects of weightlessness can be performed. Although the ISS construction was initially motivated by other factors, the station will provide an excellent opportunity for life and materials science research. The construction, maintenance and use of the international space station mark a fundamental step in the history of space flights for it provides evidence that the intense political rivalry that existed during the cold war has ceased.

As a precursor to the ISS, some degree of international cooperation had developed with manned space flights. The famous Apollo-Soyuz link-up opened the way on July 15, 1975. Twenty years later, the shuttle Discovery approached within 10 m of the Mir orbital station, close enough to allow American astronauts and their Russian counterparts to exchange hand signals through a porthole.

In March 1995, American astronaut Normann Thagard accompanied two cosmonauts aboard Soyuz-TM21 on their way to Mir. Two months later, the Atlantis shuttle carrying two Russian cosmonauts onboard docked with Mir. In June, Thagard and two Russian cosmonauts returned to Earth with Atlantis. These symbolic exchanges have reinforced the notion of international co-operation in space.

Although the human presence in space appears to be assured, the details concerning manned missions are less certain. Numerous manned flights to the moon and Mars are likely. Scientists and engineers have imagined the following possibilities:

- Lunar missions to construct permanent manned bases. Inhabitants will carry out astronomical observations outside the Earth's atmosphere and exploit the mineral deposits on the surface of the moon. Certain minerals, such as helium 3, exist in greater quantities there than on Earth. Such stations could also be the departure point for missions to Mars or to asteroids, celestial bodies from a few dozen meters to several hundred kilometers in diameter, which are found between Mars and Jupiter.
- Missions of up to two years to explore the Martian surface and potentially discover living creatures or fossils. These missions could be followed by the creation of more permanent stations where scientific and technical crews could live and work under giant domes. Certain types of research such as the creation of new molecules or microorganisms could be performed on Mars, away from potential Earth-derived contamination.

Current focus is directed toward unmanned flights, and projects for manned flights to Mars have been postponed. The Mars Pathfinder mission has demonstrated that robots can effectively explore the surface of Mars, and they will be bringing samples back to Earth in the near future. In the future, NASA plans to have robots take samples of the Martian surface. A joint French-American probe will bring these samples back to Earth in 2015 or later. If such missions find no evidence of extant or extinct life on Mars, manned flights may still need to be sent for a more thorough investigation. On the other hand, if automated missions do indicate that there is life on Mars, manned missions will certainly be considered necessary. Beyond the search for extraterrestrial life, there are other reasons for planning a manned mission to Mars. We could develop our knowledge in astronautics and propulsion technology and further our understanding of human physiology. Such a mission would unquestionably be one of humanity's great adventures in the 21st century.

Men and women will continue to explore space despite recent negative decisions. Thanks to the continued use of the Shuttle and the ISS, new names will be added to the already long list of those who have ventured into space. To date, more than 400 astronauts have flown in space and several, more than once. The duration of future manned missions will vary, but may not be as long as might be expected. Stays of three to six months are planned for ISS astronauts. Some missions, however, will require astronauts to remain in space for a much longer period, perhaps even longer than the current record. Kizim, Soloviev and Atkov lived aboard Salyut-7 for 237 consecutive days in 1984. Yuri Romenenko remained in space for 326 days and Valeri Poliakov (Figure 4), who returned to Earth on March 22, 1995, stayed for

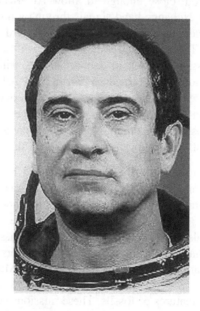

FIGURE 4 *Valeri Vladimirovitch Poliakov*
Poliakov returned to Earth after 437 days aboard the Mir station; this was the longest manned space mission. (From Institute of Biomedical Problems, Moscow.)

437 days and 18 hours aboard the Mir space station. For the female astronauts, the current record is held by the American, Shannon Lucid, who stayed 188 days onboard the Mir station in 1996 (Elena Kondokova held the previous record of 170 days).

Faced with the prospect of longer missions, the human adaptability to the extreme conditions of the space environment is a question that needs to be addressed. The answers are not simple for space has numerous physiological effects on humans, animals and plants. Space biology and medicine, two new disciplines that have developed as a result of space flights, aim at discovering these effects so that human survival can be assured in space.

3 Space: An Extreme Environment

There are a number of environmental factors that are different under space flight conditions from what we encounter here on Earth. Among these, weightlessness and exposure to cosmic radiation are the factors that have the greatest impact on living organisms, including human beings. Biologists and medical doctors are attempting to identify and understand these changes.

THE FIRST MINUTES OF A SPACE FLIGHT

From the first moments after launch and later throughout the entire mission, numerous factors affect living beings aboard a spacecraft. Some of these effects are negligible while others can cause important biological changes (Figure 5).

Inside the spacecraft, astronauts are exposed to weightlessness—the most striking environmental factor in orbital flights—as well as cosmic rays. On returning to Earth, astronauts are now exposed to lower doses of cosmic rays, but they suddenly experience gravity again.

Astronauts first experience the dynamic factors of the flight itself such as the mechanical spacecraft vibration and acceleration. The vibrations are due to the burning of fuel injected from the turbo pumps into the combustion chambers of the engines. Their magnitude can vary according to the type of spacecraft. The French astronaut, Patrick Baudry, once remarked that they were so strong that he had the impression of "sitting on the front end of a locomotive." The mechanical noise and vibrations reach their maximum intensity when the craft attains a speed of mach 1, breaks the sound barrier and leaves the Earth's atmosphere. From then on, they begin to decrease but do not cease entirely until the launcher (or booster rockets on the American Shuttle) is discarded and the engines are shut down.

Coupled with the vibrations is the acceleration produced by the launch of the spacecraft. A familiar example of this phenomenon is when a car passenger is pushed back against his seat after a sudden increase in speed. In a spacecraft, the accelerations are much greater, on the order of 3 g. At this g force level, an astronaut's body is three times heavier than normal; he is flattened against the seat and becomes unable to move. Luckily, the acceleration force generated is much lower in a modern spacecraft than in the early manned space vehicles in which the acceleration was greater than 5 g and could go as high as 8 or 10 g in a matter of seconds.

These accelerations have significant biological consequences because the cardiac system has to work harder when blood weight increases. At the same time, blood tends to get displaced in the opposite direction to the direction of movement and high g-loads can result in stomach pains, vision trouble and possible loss of consciousness.

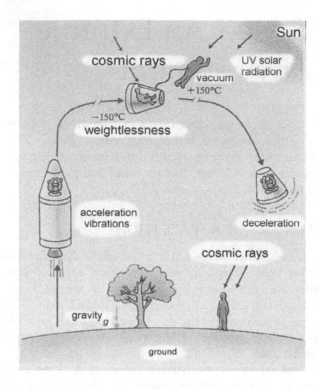

FIGURE 5 *Space environment and space flight dynamic factors*

During launch and reentry, astronauts experience strong acceleration and vibrations (space flight dynamic factors). In orbit, the space environment is characterized by a near-complete vacuum and high doses of both solar UV and cosmic rays. The temperature at the surface of the spacecraft ranges from about −150°C to +150°C depending on its position with respect to the sun.

Astronauts can avoid such effects with an anti-*g* suit, which impedes blood circulation, or through adopting an "anti-gravitational" or semi-inclined position. Aeronautical doctors, and especially those who oversee military flight personnel, also focus on these factors since people onboard these flights are subject to very high acceleration.

    Although humans can survive the dynamic factors of flight, the latter may have a negative effect on the living organisms used in sensitive experiments. For example, French scientists observed an increase in the mutation rate in Drosophila (fruit flies) aboard the Salyut space station. These results could be ascribed to cosmic rays, which have ionizing properties. Indeed X-rays or gamma rays from cobalt bombs used for cancer treatment can cause genetic mutations. However, it turned out dynamic factors were at fault since a ground-based simulation that reproduced the same vibrations resulted in the same genetic effects. Because the active phase of an experiment is performed in orbit, after vibrations and accelerations have long ceased, biologists strive to maintain their experimental material in a dormant state during takeoff to avoid such influences.

THE SPACE ENVIRONMENT
AND FLIGHT-RELATED FACTORS

Once the vibrations and acceleration have died down and the spacecraft enters into orbit, traveling at 28,000 km per hour (8 km per second), astronauts can remove their helmets and the harnesses that strap them into their seats during the launch. For the first time, they can float in the cabin. Ten minutes earlier, they were Earthlings and each movement required an effort. Now movement is easy and they experience the "ecstasy" of weightlessness. The absence of gravity, called weightlessness or microgravity (since the absence of gravity is never absolute), is a fundamental factor of space environment.

Astronauts are also exposed to a series of environmental factors. The first is temperature related. The temperature varies between −150°C and 150°C at the surface of the spacecraft depending on its position with respect to the sun. The spacecraft is slowly rotated to maintain a constant theoretical temperature of 0°C. It is also possible to stabilize a vessel in order to keep the same side facing the Earth and thus minimize temperature fluctuations. This is useful when conducting experiments in direct contact with space, i.e., in "free space." This condition was met for the LDEF (Long Duration Exposure Flight) probe on which free space experiments were performed.

The vacuum is another factor of the space environment. On the ground, humans live in an atmosphere consisting mostly of nitrogen and oxygen, at a pressure of 1 bar or 760 mmHg. As altitude increases, air becomes thinner and the atmospheric pressure rapidly decreases. At the altitude where stratospheric balloons fly, the pressure is only several thousandths of the atmospheric pressure at sea level. Satellites that orbit at an altitude varying between 250 and 400 km experience pressures less than 10^{-12} mmHg. However, atmospheric pressure is higher immediately around the spacecraft due to a slight degasification of the spacecraft outer wall. Although space is a near absolute vacuum for the biologist, it is not so for physicists. Indeed, interplanetary space still contains a few molecules such as hydrogen and small particles of meteoritic dust thousandths of a millimeter or more in diameter, which give rise to shooting stars when they come into contact with the terrestrial atmosphere.

Solar radiation is also an important factor of the space environment. Radiation is much more intense in space than on the ground because the air and atmospheric ozone do not act as a shield as they do on Earth. The sun, which is a source of constant thermonuclear reactions, emits ultraviolet light and infrared or thermal rays. UV radiation is not visible, but excessive sun exposure may cause sunburns and conjunctivitis. UV radiation also acts via the skin to transform a cholesterol-derived compound into vitamin D, thus promoting proper growth in humans. Experimentally, exposure to UV radiation has been shown to alter the structure of DNA and modify cellular genetic material. UV exposure can also induce malignant tumors such as melanoma.

Due to the intense UV cosmic radiation, the nearly absolute vacuum and the extreme temperature fluctuations, space is indeed a hostile environment. These conditions are incompatible with life in general, but there are a few organisms that can survive in such an extreme environment. Some microorganisms on Earth can form spores (cysts) displaying a remarkable resistance. Indeed, spores can survive exposure at a temperature of 100°C for several tens of minutes. The Russian scientist, Imshenentsky, found *Aspergillus* and *Penicillium* fungi at an altitude of 77 km. At that height, air is practically absent, and the temperature is around −50°C. Living bacteria have also been found on the surface of a spacecraft that had been shielded from solar radiation, even after a four-month flight. The survival record belongs without any doubt to *Streptococcus*, a bacterium that causes infections in humans. Astronauts discovered this organism in a television camera onboard Surveyor-3, a probe that had landed on the moon two and a half years earlier. It is therefore important that a spacecraft be sterilized to avoid contaminating space with bacteria that might resist the extreme conditions of a space flight.

REENTRY

A new set of environmental factors comes into play at the end of a mission, when the spaceship fires up its rockets and reenters the atmosphere. When the spacecraft reaches an altitude of 100 km, the atmospheric density begins to increase and the friction of the atmosphere against the spacecraft generates heat. To avoid a rise in temperature that would overwhelm the air-conditioning system in the cabin, vehicles are equipped with a heat shield that melts slightly as it absorbs the temperature. Thus, the heat generated by atmospheric friction during reentry is not of great concern. However, the progressive appearance of flight dynamic factors, that is the vibrations created by the deceleration of the vehicle, are a problem for astronauts. The effects of deceleration are comparable to those of acceleration, and their magnitude also depends on the spacecraft. They are more marked, for instance, on Soyuz than on the Shuttle. On Russian missions, the deceleration attains 4 *g* and can peak at 5 *g*, flattening cosmonauts against their seats. A parachute opens at an altitude of 12,000 km, but even then, if the landing were not softened during the final meters by retrorockets, cosmonauts would experience a 35-*g* acceleration.

After a spacecraft reenters the atmosphere, astronauts once again feel the weight of their arms and find it difficult to lift their hands. Upon exiting the capsule, they discover how difficult it is to walk because the stay in space has caused their bodies to "forget" gravity. Indeed, the body must suddenly readapt. Readaptation takes place without incident, but is not immediate. The French astronaut, Jean-Loup Chrétien, played tennis at the Star City training center outside Moscow before his flight aboard Salyut-7 in 1982. After the seven-day mission, he felt healthy enough to play tennis the day following his return to Baikonur, but he kept missing the ball and soon found it impossible to continue the match. The incident is easy to explain: the vestibular apparatus—the nervous center responsible for balance and movement coordination—was unable to engage the precise reflexes needed for hitting the ball on a tennis court. Twenty-four hours later, however, he had completely readapted to gravity and was back to normal.

In conclusion, many factors can affect human beings during a space flight. However, the spaceship cabin provides protection from the environmental hazards such as vacuum conditions and temperature variations. The cabin is maintained at about 20°C, and its atmosphere is similar to that on Earth. This was not the case on the earlier Apollo flights, where cabins were filled with oxygen at a pressure equal to a third of that on Earth. Astronauts are also completely protected from UV radiation by the cabin lining. During an EVA, an astronaut's spacesuit protects him from free space. However, he will still be exposed—as he is inside the cabin—to weightlessness and cosmic radiation, the intensity of which is much greater in space than on Earth.

SPACE BIOLOGY AND MEDICINE

The first objective of space biology and space medicine is to ensure astronauts' survival. This issue seems to have been resolved given that more than 400 men and women have flown into space safely and, barring a few exceptions, are all in good health. Some have even been able to live for many months in weightlessness. Yet survival in space is far from being completely under control in that microgravity causes serious physiological stress. The human body compensates for the stress induced thanks to its remarkable regulatory systems. However, the influence of microgravity over very long space flights is unknown. A mission to Mars would last approximately two years, interrupted by a stay of several months on the planet itself, and the subsequent colonization of space would require that several generations follow one another in a spaceship. It is unknown whether cosmic radiation might induce inherited genetic mutations in offspring born on such long missions. Fundamental research will improve current knowledge little by little, and the Skylab and Soviet space station programs have certainly played a very important part in this respect. A large space station will require the development of new life supporting techniques. One possible system involves using living organisms capable of absorbing carbon dioxide to renew the atmosphere. Living organisms might also be used to produce proteins and sugars as food for the astronauts. Such techniques are under study in the American CELSS program (controlled ecological life support system), but first it will be essential to understand the effects of weightlessness and cosmic rays on organisms that are to be used in space.

The second objective of space biology and medicine is less practical than the first. Gravity and cosmic rays are two factors of the environment that have a constant impact on all living beings: species were created, developed and evolved in their presence. An understanding of their effects is of major importance in fundamental biology and physiology. Indeed, space provides remarkable and unique study conditions as it "cancels out" the effects of gravity over an extended period of time and exposes living beings to higher doses of cosmic radiation than on Earth. This is precisely the sort of situation a biologist might wish for. When a biologist wants to understand the influence of a particular vitamin, he induces an avitaminosis, or vitamin deficiency, so that he might study what happens when the vitamin is absent from the organism under study. Conversely, he will wish to induce a hypervitaminosis to study the effects of vitamin overdose. Similarly, specialists in biology and medicine can exploit the absence of gravity in space flights to run experiments under weightlessness and compare them with Earth-based hypergravity experiments.

Ensuring the survival of humans in space and understanding the effects of gravity and cosmic radiation are the main objectives of space life science. Another field, known as exobiology, has to do with the search for extraterrestrial life forms. The last chapter will deal with exobiology.

4 Gravity and Weightlessness

Gravity is an invisible force that has a constant effect upon the terrestrial environment, causing rivers to empty into oceans and keeping objects on the surface of the planet. Weightlessness—that is, the absence of gravity—is one of the most striking aspects of a space flight. It alters an astronaut's motor performance and lifestyle and gives rise to a whole series of physiological stress responses. These are usually discrete though some can be more striking. A quick summary of the physics of weightlessness and how it is generated in space will lead to a better understanding of these effects.

GALILEO AND NEWTON

If an object such as a rock is dropped, it falls vertically to the ground. If the same rock is thrown in a horizontal direction, it follows a curved or parabolic trajectory before landing. The greater the force, the further away it will land. Subjected to a huge initial velocity, it could orbit the Earth in a circular trajectory as an artificial satellite. For this to happen, the rock would have to be accelerated to 7.91 km per second (17,000 mph), which is known as the first cosmic speed. A satellite launched by a rocket travelling at this speed enters into a circular or elliptical orbit. With an even greater force, an object can overcome the Earth's gravity and become a space probe.

Greek philosophers argued that objects fall to be reunited with their natural physical place, the Earth. According to Aristotle, the heavier the object, the faster it falls. It was not until the 16th century that a major scientific breakthrough was made when Galileo discovered that objects fell with increasing rather than constant speed: regardless of weight or size, all objects fall with the same acceleration. However, this only holds true in a vacuum. Under normal conditions, air resistance also increases with speed. When the air resistance becomes equal to the weight of a falling object, the latter falls at a constant speed. This is what happens to skydivers before opening their parachutes: several divers falling at the same speed can join up, separate and rejoin. Galileo's observations and the laws he formulated after dropping objects off the tower of Pisa were so revolutionary that he was ordered to stop teaching. In 1633, a tribunal of the Inquisition condemned him to live in a guarded residence near Florence where he died nine years later, in 1642, still sequestered by the Inquisition.

The atmosphere in England was very different. In 1666, the English physicist Robert Hooke had already put forth the idea of a central attractive force between celestial bodies. The English astronomer Edmund Halley gave an explanation of the structure of the universe based on the existence of an attractive force between stars that was proportional to their mass. Isaac Newton had the genius to pursue this idea further. Newton published his *Principia Mathematica Philosophiae Naturalis* (Mathematical Principles of Natural Philosophy) in 1687, 45 years after Galileo's death, when he was a 25-year-old student at Cambridge. His 500-page treatise in Latin explained Galileo's theories and made a fundamental contribution to the laws of physics and astronomy. When he died in 1727, he was honored with a funeral worthy of royalty.

Legend has it that Newton found the inspiration for his Universal Law in Woolsthorpe, Lincolnshire where he happened to observe an apple fall from a tree. According to this law, all objects exert a force on all other objects; the magnitude of this attraction depends on the mass of the objects and is inversely proportional to the square of the distance between their centers. This principle applies to all objects, regardless of size or density. Falling rocks and apples as well as stars and planets exhibit a gravitational force. Thus, the sun attracts the planets into orbit around itself, and the planets attract all objects in contact with them. The gravitational force—designated by the symbol g—is never repulsive like electric or magnetic forces. It is an attractive force that causes all free-falling objects to accelerate toward Earth (in the absence of air).

Thus gravity attracts all objects toward the center of the Earth and is the origin of their weight. Weight is defined as the product of the mass of an object times g, where mass is the quantity of matter that an object contains. The mass of a given object is constant and independent of its physical location. Gravity, on the other hand, is not a constant value. The mass of the Earth is 6.10^{24} kg, and its resulting gravity is 9.8 m/s^{-2}. The Earth being ellipsoidal and slightly flattened near the poles, gravity varies with latitude, albeit very weakly. Other celestial bodies with a mass different from that of the Earth will have different g values. For the moon, $g = 1.52$ m/s^{-2}, which corresponds to 1/6 of terrestrial gravity. In other words, a person weighing 60 kg on Earth will weigh only 10 kg on the moon. On Mars, also less massive than the Earth, g is about 4 m/s^{-2}.

Objects exert a force on the Earth. However, because the mass of the Earth is considerably greater than that of any object on its surface, the terrestrial attractive force is dominant. Human beings remain anchored to the planet's surface, regardless of their geographical location! Any falling object falls to Earth toward its center of gravity. The law of gravity is universal and applies to all celestial bodies; this law explains the movement of stars in relation to each other as well as the attraction of dust particles until they come to form planets. According to the recent theory of quantum gravitation, gravity also acts upon the smallest particles of matter, which are separated by distances of less than a millionth of a billionth of a billionth of a centimeter! Gravity is present throughout the universe and is responsible for curving space according to theories of relativity. Yet while its effects can be observed every day, its nature remains mysterious.

FREE-FALL AND SPACE FLIGHTS

The Earth constantly pulls human beings and all objects toward it, giving rise to body weight. The pull of gravity is only blocked by the fact that the ground is solid. In soft ground, such as swampland or quicksand, an individual begins to sink and

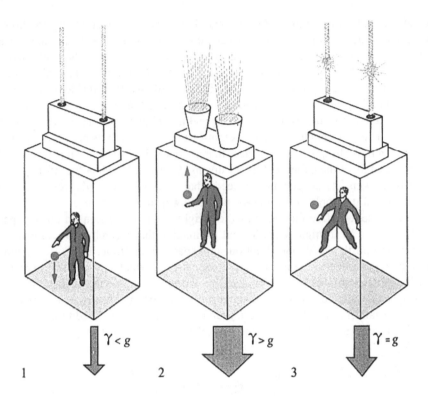

$\gamma < g$ 1

$\gamma > g$ 2

$\gamma = g$ 3

FIGURE 6 *How can free-fall and weightlessness be explained?*

A man in an upright position is inside a lift. Suppose a vacuum is created in the lift shaft. Under usual gravity conditions, the acceleration of a falling body is 10 m/s^{-2}, that is, much higher than the acceleration of the lift going down; the passenger therefore remains "stuck" to the floor of the lift cabin.

When the lift is pushed down by rockets, its acceleration exceeds that of gravity with the result that the passenger and the apple go up towards the ceiling of the lift cabin.

Supposing the lift cable is broken, the lift, the passenger and any object in the cabin are now exposed to the attractive force of the Earth and have the same acceleration. They are therefore in free-fall. Both the passenger and the ball can now float since they are under weightlessness.

becomes aware of this pull. If all obstacles and supports are removed, an object will fall vertically with a uniform acceleration along a linear path. The object will free-fall with an acceleration of 9.81 m/s^{-2}. To understand what free-fall and weightlessness are, let us consider a man standing in a lift cabin with opaque walls (Figure 6). Under normal running conditions when the lift goes down suspended to cables, the acceleration of the moving cabin is less than the acceleration of gravity.

The passenger is therefore still submitted to the Earth's attraction and stays "stuck" to the floor of the cabin. If he lets a ball drop from his hand, it will fall as usual toward the floor. Let us now suppose we create a vacuum inside the lift cabin and the lift shaft, and that we cut the cables. The cabin and its passenger are no longer stopped by any obstacles and, therefore, start to free-fall. An observer situated on the outside of the lift shaft (supposing the walls were transparent) will note that the cabin is indeed free-falling. On the other hand, the passenger, unable to observe the outside world, will not be aware of any movement. As he falls at the same speed and acceleration as the cabin, his feet will come off the floor of the cabin and he will start to float freely; simple movements will allow him to move toward the walls or the roof of the cabin. If he lets go of a ball, it will also float inside the cabin. As they are moving with an acceleration of 9.81 m/s⁻², the force of gravity will be cancelled, and the weight of the passenger and any objects present in the cabin will disappear. They are said to be under weightlessness. Although its effects on the man in the cabin have disappeared, it is clear that gravity still exists since it is responsible for the free-fall of the cabin and its occupants. Conversely, when the lift is pushed down by rockets, its acceleration exceeds that of gravity with the result that the passenger and the apple go up toward the ceiling of the lift cabin.

The concept of free-fall explains the weightlessness experienced during space flights (Figure 7). It might seem logical to imagine that a satellite would abandon its orbit around the Earth and shoot out into space at any time. However, satellites are held in orbit due to the Earth's gravitational pull, which causes them to continuously "fall" toward the Earth. The satellite remains in orbit due to the initial thrust of its rocket motors upon launch and the resulting inertia. As there is no air resistance, it is in constant free-fall and, as a result, under weightlessness. In addition, satellites experience uniform circular movement. As explained by Newton, this type of movement

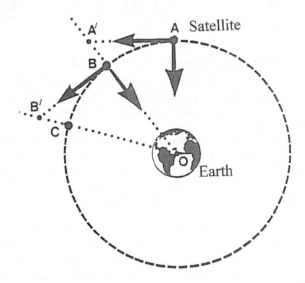

FIGURE 7 *Free-fall and weightlessness (a simplified explanation)*

Supposing a satellite is moving in a circular orbit around the Earth. At point A, it is submitted to two perpendicular forces: gravity and the force of inertia created by the thrust of the rocket during the launch. After a short time, the satellite will reach A' from the push given by the force of inertia. However, it is simultaneously exposed to gravity, so that it "goes" from A' to B. It is all the time in free-fall. The satellite is under weightlessness and remains in a circular orbit under the influence of gravity.

Newton had already shown that the moon is at all times "falling down" toward the Earth.

consists of a linear movement at a constant speed caused by inertia associated with a uniformly accelerated movement, orientated toward the Earth's center and caused by gravity. If only the linear movement is taken into account, it can be said that satellites move at a constant speed.

KONSTANTIN TSIOLKOVSKY AND JULES VERNE

The weightlessness of space flights was imagined many years before Yuri Gagarin's flight and even before the first Sputnik was launched.

The Soviet mathematician Konstantin Tsiolkovsky (1857–1935) was the first to speculate that gravity would "disappear" during a space flight (Figure 8). Tsiolkovsky was a teacher in a private high school in Kaluga, a small town 200 km from Moscow. His studies on propulsion reaction led him to play an essential role in the development of astronautics. He outlined the importance of several-stage rockets, the use of liquid oxygen hydrogen as fuel, and international cooperation for interplanetary travel. In a letter written 50 years before Gagarin's flights, he speculated that the human race would not remain forever on Earth but would "pursue light and space and would go beyond the limits of the atmosphere to conquer all that revolves around the sun." He also imagined the state of weightlessness in space flights, as his remarkable drawings displayed in the space museum in Kaluga illustrate. He worked

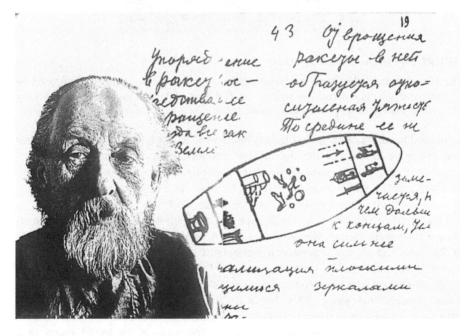

FIGURE 8 *Tsiolkovsky (1857–1935)*

A pioneer in astronautics, he carried out many studies on rocket propulsion. He described what happens when a man is exposed to weightlessness and understood the importance of international cooperation in the conquest of space. (From Institute of Biomedical Problems, Moscow.)

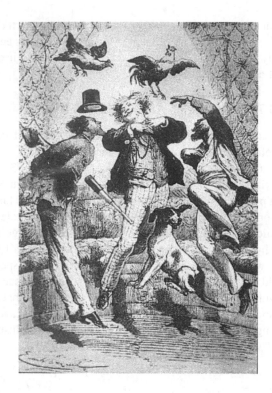

FIGURE 9 *From the Earth to the Moon*

The French writer Jules Verne imagined the state of "inebriation" (a term often used by astronauts) of men in a state of weightlessness. However he thought that weightlessness only occurred at the Lagrange point, when Earth's force of gravity is cancelled by lunar gravity.

alone and his theories remained largely unknown. It was not until many years later that his achievement became universally recognized. In 1918, he was elected a member of the Socialist Academy, later the Soviet Academy of Sciences, and received a state pension from the People's Commissar. The space museum was built in his hometown in recognition of his pioneering work.

Even before Tsiolkovsky, the French science fiction writer Jules Verne, well known for novels such as *Voyage to the Centre of the Earth* and *Around the World in 80 Days*, had already described the effects of weightlessness in *From the Earth to the Moon*, published in 1865 (Figure 9).

In this novel, the passengers aboard the ship Colombia (a rather coincidental name) venture into space. They begin to float freely once terrestrial and lunar attractions cancel each other out. This is scientifically inaccurate, since we now know that weightlessness is a dynamic factor appearing in the initial stages of a space flight and persisting throughout the flight, regardless of the distance between the craft and the Earth. However, Verne also described the space travelers as being "drunk"; he had foreseen the inebriation of space, a term so often used by astronauts.

In addition, there are three points to be made. First, the strength of Earth's gravity depends on the distance of an object from the center of the Earth. When climbing a mountain, for example, g decreases. Second, at an altitude of 300 km, the average space flight altitude, g is reduced by only 10 percent. Third, even if the distance from the Earth were greater, this factor alone would not create weightlessness, since it is a dynamic phenomenon which appears only when a spacecraft is in free-fall.

SIMULATING AND CREATING WEIGHTLESSNESS ON EARTH

Given the high cost of space flights, attempts have been made to reproduce microgravity on Earth artificially. On this point, it is worth noting that vacuum and weightlessness are sometimes confused. In fact, the two factors are very different, and while a vacuum can easily be produced on Earth, the weightlessness experienced in space cannot be duplicated on Earth except for very short times. Only simulation techniques are used in most cases.

The most common technique for space flight simulation uses specially designed large planes that can fly with parabolic trajectories (Figure 10). These planes, which fly at high altitudes, dive and climb again at great speed. When they do this, there is a brief moment of microgravity at the end of the ascending phase of the trajectory. The weightlessness produced under these conditions allows the crew to float in the cabin as if they were in a spaceship. Unfortunately, the duration of weightlessness is only approximately 20 seconds. To increase the exposure time, 40 to 50 successive rounds with this parabolic pattern are usually performed. Each period of weightlessness is preceded by acceleration and followed by deceleration phases when crewmembers

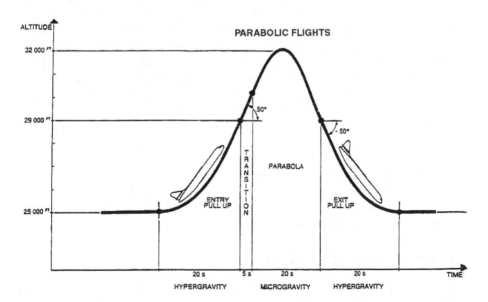

FIGURE 10 *Parabolic flights*

At the end of the ascending phase of the aircraft trajectory, the passengers do not experience any acceleration and are in weightlessness for 20 to 25 seconds.

experience gravitational levels of about 1.8 g. As early as 1961, an American scientist named T.L. Jahn devised an interesting biological experiment in which a culture of *Tetrahymena* protozoa was placed aboard a parabolic flight. Under normal gravitational conditions, these single-cell organisms tend to form a cluster in the culture medium, forming sinewy-shaped clouds. Interestingly, these clouds disappeared in weightlessness and reappeared as soon as the plane completed its parabolic flight. Jahn thus demonstrated for the first time that gravity exerts an influence on cells.

Another technique, developed in Germany, consists of releasing a capsule from a balloon at an altitude of 30 to 45 km. The free-fall of the capsule lasts 20 to 60 seconds and exposes the payload inside it to a microgravity equal to one thousandth of gravity (10^{-3} g). Drop towers are another means of generating microgravity. There are drop towers in the United States, France and Italy, but the most remarkable tower is the one in Bremen, Germany. It features a "drop chamber" that is 110 m high and 3.5 cm in diameter. A loaded capsule is dropped in the chamber, falling at a speed of 160 km per hour. A collection of pumps with a total air output of 30,000 m³/h creates a vacuum inside the chamber. A microgravity of about 10^{-4} g (0.0001 g) is thus obtained in the tower. It is a remarkable feat, but of limited interest to biologists since the microgravity conditions last a maximum of eight seconds.

Weightlessness can also be produced using rocket probes, which rise vertically in order to have a suborbital trajectory. These rocket probes were actually the first spacecraft. As early as the 13th century, the Chinese military used what they called "fire arrows" based on the same propulsion principles. Current developments in rocketry go back to Tsiolkovsky's theoretical calculations on the flight, launch speed and fuel consumption of rockets. Werner von Braun later perfected the V-2 rocket for the German war effort. After relocating to the United States, he developed new engines for scientific research and for launching space vehicles. Rocket probes are now widely used to study atmospheric physics, as they easily reach the mesosphere situated an altitude between 50 and 85 km, where the ozone layer filters ultraviolet radiation. They can also reach the ionosphere and the exosphere beyond 300 km. Biologists use these rockets since they can achieve a microgravity on the order of 10^{-3} to 10^{-4} g. It is for this reason that the Americans and the Soviets used them before manned flights. In the early 1950s the French biologist Robert Grandpierre and his colleagues placed a monkey fitted with electrodes in order to record its electroencephalogram in each of two rockets. They later repeated their experiment using a rat.

Ballistic missiles achieve microgravity for only several minutes, yet they continue to be regularly used by the European Space Agency for studying the influence of microgravity on rapid phenomena like fertilization or the binding of chemical compounds to cell membrane receptors.

SIMULATING MICROGRAVITY

Drop towers, parabolic flights and rocket probes are the only means available for duplicating weightlessness outside space flights. All other techniques produce only some of the effects of weightlessness. One way to simulate the effects of microgravity on biological models is immobilization. Under normal circumstances, changes in body position increase or decrease the influence of gravity on the body, which in turn affects the interplay of complex regulatory systems. Prolonged immobilization in a horizontal position reduces the effects of the gravitational force on the cardiovascular system, on muscle, as well as on bones since the latter carry the weight of the body in the upright position.

Antiorthostatic hypokinesia, also known as bed rest, is the most commonly used method to simulate microgravity. A person is confined to bed with a head-down tilt of 6 degrees for several hours, days or even weeks. The record is held by two subjects who remained in bed for one year in a Moscow laboratory. Antiorthostatic hypokinesia allows the physiological responses to be studied throughout the experiment, while during a space flight, the first measurements are usually taken up to two days after launch. Astronauts are also subject to a lengthy prelaunch immobilization. Bed rest can be used to develop countermeasures that might decrease the effects of weightlessness during and after the flight. The usefulness of hypokinetic studies has been demonstrated for the cardiovascular system, bone and muscle. However, the effects of space flights on balance cannot be reproduced with hypokinesis. Indeed, the weight of the otoliths in the vestibular apparatus is not modified, and the subject obviously cannot move about as astronauts do in space.

Another simulation method is water immersion where subjects wear a space suit in a swimming pool. When an object is immersed in liquid, it is subjected to a vertical push equal to the weight of the liquid displaced. Astronauts training in a swimming pool can therefore move with greater ease. This technique is currently used to simulate EVAs and to allow astronauts to practice maneuvers they will have to perform in space. Keeping the head above water for an extended period of time is a similar technique. Under these conditions, the pressure created by water on the lower limbs and the abdomen results in a rapid fluid shift toward the thoracic region and the head. However, problems related to hygiene and thermal control have led to the use of other techniques.

For instance, specific body parts can be immobilized. This technique is used primarily with animals for muscle and skeletal research. Cutting a tendon or motor nerve puts the corresponding muscle or group of muscles at rest. Wearing a cast causes muscular atrophy and decalcification, both of which are also observed in weightlessness. An imaginative although somewhat controversial technique for recreating this type of "unloading" is the suspended rat technique designed by Emily Morey-Holton of NASA in 1979 and later modified by E.A. Il'yim, Chief of Scientific Programs for the Soviet biosatellite program. A rat is equipped with a harness linked to a pulley system that allows it to move about the cage (Figure 11). The apparatus can also be fixed directly to the tail. The rat is thus suspended in a head-down position at a 30-degree angle, resting only on its forelimbs, while remaining free to turn 360 degrees and search the entire surface of its cage for food. The animal rapidly adapts to the harness. This technique simulates the effects of weightlessness in bones and muscles of the hind legs. It also allows changes in blood flow to be simulated since, as in the case of humans under weightlessness, the blood of suspended rats tends to shift toward head and thorax.

Rapid and slow clinostats—rotating discs on which a biological organism can be placed for study—are also used. The German scientist Wolfgang Briegleb invented the rapid clinostat. This device allows culture cells placed in a small glass

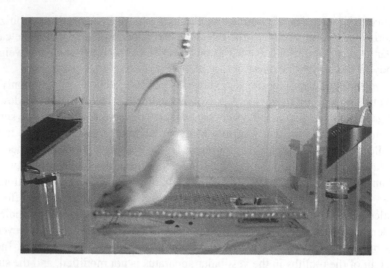

FIGURE 11 *Microgravity simulation*

A rat is equipped with a harness and suspended upside down, resting only on its forelegs. Microgravity effects can thus be simulated in bones and muscles of the hind-legs. (Laboratory of Physiology, Lyon, France.)

tube filled with liquid to be attached onto a platform that rotates at 100 rpm. The combined action of the centrifugal force, gravity and the viscosity of the medium causes the cells to "float" when they are in the horizontal rotation axis, as if they were in a state of weightlessness or microgravity. In such experiments, the small granules or amyloplasts of statocytes—cells located in plant roots—no longer have the tendency to precipitate. They float in the cytoplasm and behave as they do on a space flight. The rapid clinostat thus provides interesting results, and many European scientists go to Bonn in the hope of confirming the results of their space experiments or perfecting research projects intended for future missions. With the slow clinostat, invented by T.A. Knight in England in 1806, a plant is attached to a support turning at approximately one revolution per minute around a horizontal axis. With such a device, the effects of gravity are periodically reversed as the plant either has a normal orientation, i.e., with the roots pointing downward, or the opposite orientation with the roots pointing upward. Today's clinostats are often more complex and can rotate in different planes. These instruments are mainly used to investigate geotropism, which is the study of the response of plants to gravity. More recently, biologists have used a random positioning machine developed by Fokker Space in the Netherlands. This machine usually gives a better simulation of microgravity since objects are successively orientated in three different planes.

In conclusion, certain techniques allow weightlessness to be simulated on Earth but over too brief a time for most biological and medical experiments. Others simulate weightlessness by reducing or altering some of the effects of gravity. Because these techniques have limitations, it is clear that space is a new and irreplaceable laboratory allowing one to study the effects of weightlessness and, consequently, those of gravity on the living world.

5 Physiological and Biological Effects of Weightlessness in Humans and Animals

The Cardiovascular System

The first responses to weightlessness, which are more acute for some individuals than for others, come into play once the spacecraft enters into orbit and the astronauts remove their pressurized suits. The face becomes congested, and astronauts experience a floating sensation. Other symptoms soon appear as each cell, tissue and organ are submitted to the influence of weightlessness. The cardiovascular, musculoskeletal and vestibular systems are the most affected, which is not surprising given that gravity has an important effect on all three.

The cardiovascular system was of great concern to the engineers and physicians preparing for manned space flights in both the Soviet Union and the United States from the earliest days of astronautics. This concern was well founded because by eliminating the weight of blood, weightlessness might cause significant disturbances to the cardiovascular system and to cardiac activity in particular. Ground simulation experiments provided interesting clues but did not allow one to ascertain if an astronaut's cardiovascular system could adapt to the absence of gravity. Before sending humans into space, it was imperative to learn whether living beings could survive a space flight. Thus, began a series of experiments using animals.

THE FIRST AMERICAN TESTS

Even before Gagarin's flight, studies were carried out on numerous launches, which nevertheless represent only a fraction of the enormous effort made in the early days of space flights. Indeed rockets and space cabins needed to be perfected. Devices necessary for the nutrition and respiration of the living beings on these flights had to be devised. The development of radiotelemetry was also required to inform ground control centers of a biological subject's state of health during the space flight, and reentry techniques allowing safe recovery had to be designed. Although these endeavors were often crowned with success, certain experiments were disappointing while others ended tragically, and the animals whose sacrifice was necessary for the development of astronautics should not be forgotten.

After a series of rocket flights containing monkeys and mice that were never recovered, the United States carried out its first "successful" flight in September 1951, when a Rhesus monkey and 11 mice flew aboard the Aerobee-2 probe. The monkey's electrocardiogram, arterial and venous pressures were recorded, and cameras photographed the mice's movements to study their motor activity. All the animals were recovered, but the monkey died immediately. The Aerobee-3 probe flight of May 1952 with two Cebus monkeys and two mice aboard was a perfect success, and in April 1958, a probe containing mice reached an altitude of 160 km but this time, the animals were not recovered. In December of the same year, a squirrel monkey was placed aboard the Bioflight-1 probe. This animal is an interesting biological model because it never drinks, drawing water only from ingested food. Its temperature and cardiac rhythm were recorded as the rocket reached an altitude of 186 km. The little monkey resisted weightlessness successfully, but never returned to Earth. In May of the following year, two rhesus monkeys and a squirrel monkey were placed aboard Bioflight-2, but the telemetry system failed as soon as the probe was launched. However, recovery occurred normally, and the animals were found to have well tolerated the flight.

In October 1960, the Atlas rocket, which was later to be widely used by the United States, had reached a stage of perfection that allowed it to pass through the recently discovered Van Allan belts—the radiation phenomenon surrounding the Earth. The probe was unable to attain orbit, but the capsule was recovered. The three mice aboard had tolerated the exposure to cosmic radiation, and the offspring they were to have were normal. Obviously overoptimistic conclusions about exposure to cosmic radiation cannot be drawn from these results, and we shall see that radiation should be treated with caution. In January 1961, the United States further prepared for the first human space flight by putting a chimpanzee in the seat that would soon be occupied by Alan Shepard in the Mercury capsule on May 5, 1961. Respiration, electrocardiogram and temperature were recorded, and NASA was reassured when the chimpanzee was recovered in good health. However, it was only a ballistic flight.

Although Alan Shepard's flight and later, Virgil Grissom's were successful, this did not spell an end to animal experiments since the effects of long-term exposure to weightlessness were still unknown. In February 1962, a monkey made an orbital flight lasting 183 minutes aboard the Mercury capsule and was recovered safe and sound. After the failure of the first satellite flight dedicated entirely to biology in 1966 and the successful flight of Biosatellite-2 in which single-cell organisms, plants and insects were subjected to weightlessness for 48 hours, the Americans wanted to break new ground with Biosatellite-3 in June 1969. A macaque named Bonny was fitted with probes to measure its arterial pressure, cardiac rhythm and brain temperature, and record its electroencephalogram. The flight lasted nearly 9 days, but Bonny died of stress shortly after recovery. The excessive number of probes and electrodes and a lack of preparation to stress had not sufficiently prepared the animal for the experiment. Many years passed before the United States once again considered studying the effects of weightlessness on monkeys in spite of them being an interesting biological model because of the similarity between their cardiovascular system and ours.

THE FIRST SOVIET TESTS

Efforts similar to those in the United States were being carried out even earlier in the Soviet Union. Between 1949 and 1952, nine dogs flew aboard rockets that reached the modest altitude of 100 km and their pulse rate, arterial pressure and respiratory rate were recorded. The same measurements were made on nine dogs in 1957 but this time, the rockets reached an altitude of 200 km. Then, Laika became the first mammal to circle the Earth on November 3, 1957 aboard Sputnik-2. Telemetry indicated that the dog endured the flight well but Laika suffocated due to oxygen depletion. Recovery had not been thought possible at the time. It is important to remember that Laïka's historic flight took place only one month after the launch of Sputnik-1.

Between 1958 and 1959, 4 ballistic flights were launched carrying 4 dogs and a rabbit. This time recovery had been planned and was successful. The fourth Sputnik flight with a dog took place on May 15, 1960. The electrocardiogram showed normal cardiac function, but the dog was not recovered. On August 20, 1960, an entire menagerie with 2 dogs, 42 mice, rats and Drosophila flies as well as plant seeds were launched and recovered 24 hours later. Another orbital flight with 2 dogs onboard Sputnik-6 took place in December 1960 using the Korabl-3 rocket. The telemetry system functioned normally, but the capsule and the dogs burned up during reentry into the atmosphere. In 1961, the flights of Korabl-4 and -5 were successful and the hearts of the dogs resisted well. Eighteen days later, Gagarin would launch himself into the cosmos with the assurance for which he was famous. At first glance, preliminary experiments seemed to show that the cardiovascular system could withstand the effects of weightlessness. In fact, it turns out a space flight causes numerous disturbances. Brief information about the cardiovascular system and how it is influenced by gravity will provide a better understanding of these disturbances.

BASIC CONCEPTS IN PHYSIOLOGY

The cardiovascular system consists of the arterial system, which is a high pressure system that terminates with the capillaries in the organs (Figure 12). The venous system is a low pressure system that starts in the organs and transports blood through the vena cava and into the right auricle or atrium of the heart. The blood then flows toward the right ventricle and reaches the lungs via the pulmonary artery. The pulmonary veins bring the blood back to the heart (left auricle). The blood is squeezed into the left ventricle and leaves the heart through the aorta. The aorta and its branches carry the blood to all parts of the body. Oxygen, water and nutrients cross the capillary walls and are delivered to the cells. Venous blood contains CO_2 and metabolism waste products created by cellular activity. The kidneys eliminate a significant amount of this waste.

It is important to recall that the kidney is made up of small tubules called nephrons. Nephrons terminate at the collecting tubes that lead to the pelvis and are

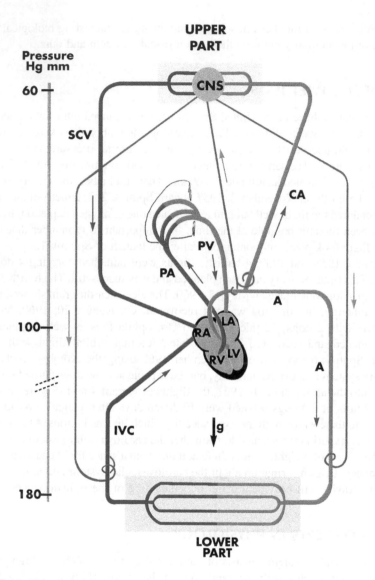

FIGURE 12 *The cardiovascular system (see Color figure I at the end of the book)*

Nerve impulses originate from nerve endings around the arch of the aorta and the point where the internal carotid artery starts. In response, nerve impulses control the diameter of peripheral vessels thereby altering blood flow. The right ventricle sends the deoxygenated blood to the lungs. The left ventricle pumps the oxygenated blood into the aorta and its branches. The effect of gravity is different in the upper and lower parts of the body.

CNS: Central Nervous System
SVC: Superior vena cava
CA: Carotid Artery
PV: Pulmonary Vein
PA: Pulmonary Artery
RA: Right Atrium
RV: Right Ventricle
LA: Left Atrium
LV: Left Ventricle
A: Aorta
IVC: Inferior vena cava

connected to the bladder by the two ureters. The blind extremity of nephrons is slightly inflated to form the glomeruli. Each glomerulus has a central hollow containing a tuft of blood capillaries that filter the water, urea, and mineral salts passing through their membranes and into the lumen of nephrons. A large quantity of useful substances is subsequently absorbed through the nephron wall and returns to the bloodstream, while the remainder forms the urine.

This absorption function is under the influence of regulatory systems because urinary excretion, like liquid intake, must adapt to body needs. Two hormones ensure this kidney regulation: the antidiuretic hormone, or ADH, and aldosterone. ADH, also known as vasopressin, is synthesised by the neuronal cells of the hypothalamic nuclei in the brain. The hormone then passes into the bloodstream and is stored in the posterior lobe of the pituitary gland. Aldosterone is secreted by the adrenal gland cortex, which forms the outer part of the adrenal gland. This region is itself regulated by different factors and in particular by the renin-angiotensin system. Renin is synthesised in the kidneys by the glomeruli blood capillaries. It is responsible for the transformation of a liver-derived precursor into angiotensin in the blood. This in turn stimulates the secretion of aldosterone. Vasopressin and aldosterone control urinary excretion, vasopressin tending to increase the absorption of water—hence its diuretic activity—whereas aldosterone stimulates sodium absorption. Urine, therefore, does not have the same composition as the glomerular filtrate (Figure 13).

For many years it was thought that vasopressin and aldosterone were the only hormones involved in the regulation of diuresis. However, there is in fact another regulatory hormone synthesised in the heart itself, and its discovery created quite a stir. The heart, until recently considered to be nothing more than a pump ensuring blood circulation, turns out to be an endocrine gland as well. The myocardium fibers or cardiac muscle cells are indeed very similar to the striated muscular fibers that form the skeletal muscles such as biceps and leg muscles. Yet certain myocardium cells situated in the auricle walls have a special structure: they not only contain myofibrils, which are responsible for their contraction, but also a large quantity of small granules that are visible in the electron microscope. These granules contain atrial natriuretic peptide (ANP), a hormone which affects the regulation of arterial pressure, blood mass and diuresis, and which has an impact on the cardiovascular system of astronauts as we shall see.

THE EFFECTS OF GRAVITY

It is now important to understand the effects of gravity on the cardiovascular system of human beings living under normal conditions on Earth. Gravity creates the weight of the blood mass and thus affects the entire vascular system. Its influence evidently depends on the part of the body under consideration and its orientation. In an upright position, gravity causes blood pressure in the vessels situated under the heart to be greater than the intra-cardiac pressure. If the arterial pressure is 100 mmHg (mercury) at heart level, it is 200 mmHg in the arteries in the feet and only 60 mmHg in the vessels of the head. In the vertical position, gravity forces the blood to the body's lower extremities but hinders the flow of arterial blood to the brain. When moving

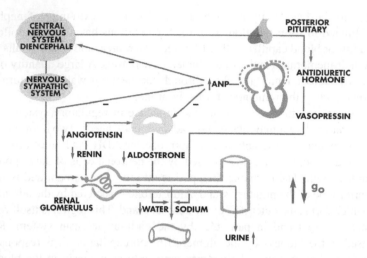

FIGURE 13 *A summary of proposed physiological responses to weightlessness (see Color figure II at the end of the book)*

In space, exposure to microgravity results in:

1. A decrease, which not always observed, in the antidiuretic hormone vasopressin. This hormone is secreted by the diencephalon in the brain and stored in the posterior lobe of the hypophysis.

2. An increase in the secretion of the atrial natriuretic hormone by the heart.

3. A lowering in the secretion of angiotensin and renin, which control the synthesis of aldosterone by the adrenal glands.

4. These changes provoke a loss in fluids by resorption of water and salt (sodium and potassium) in the nephrons (in the kidney). Water and salts from blood pass through the renal glomeruli.

It should be pointed out that results vary considerably for different flights and according to the time when the samples were obtained. Furthermore, a large part of this diagram is based on simulation experiments carried out on Earth. (Laboratory of Physiology, Lyon, France.)

from a horizontal position to an upright position, the blood tends to accumulate in the lower part of the body due to its weight, resulting in decreased pressure in the arteries situated above the heart. This hypotension will have repercussions on baroreceptors located in the walls of the internal carotid artery immediately above its point of origin, an area called the carotid sinus.

The impulses from the baroreceptors usually inhibit the nerves that cause the narrowing of blood vessels (vasoconstriction) and slow down cardiac rhythm. When moving from a supine to an upright position, the aorta wall and the carotid sinus are less distended. Because the baroreceptors are less stimulated, their braking action is also diminished and this causes a vasoconstriction reflex, particularly in the smaller arteries, as well as an increase in the cardiac rate. Due to these regulatory phenomena, arterial pressure can be maintained, and the accumulation of blood in the lower extremities can be limited. This is not the same under weightlessness, which causes important modifications in the cardiovascular system.

Change in blood mass distribution

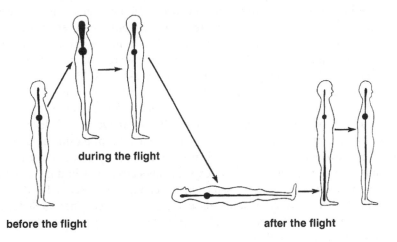

during the flight

before the flight   after the flight

FIGURE 14 *Diagrams of fluid movement in a human body*

1. On Earth, in the supine position, blood and other fluids are evenly distributed due to the regulation of blood circulation.

2. In space, fluids move toward the upper part of the body because the downward force of gravity is absent. The blood flow regulating system tends to be at rest.

3. As a result of an adaptation process and fluid loss, a decrease in fluid redistribution occurs.

4. On returning to Earth, the regulatory system is still at rest and, for a short time, gravity pulls the blood downward when the person moves from a supine to a standing position (deconditioning).

THE FIRST EFFECTS OF WEIGHTLESSNESS

In the absence of a hydrostatic force generated by gravity at the onset of the orbital phase of a space flight, 0.6 to 2 litres of blood and interstitial fluid leave the lower part of the body and drain towards the thoracic, cervical and cephalic regions (Figure 14). This fluid movement explains the commonly observed bloating of an astronaut's face, known as "puffy face," the sensation of heaviness in the head and the nasal congestion while neck and hand veins appear distended. Conversely, leg volume decreases, a phenomenon referred to as "bird legs." As soon as these responses were known, it was thought that the body would react in space as it had in ground simulation experiments such as bed rest and water immersion. Under these conditions, a blood and interstitial fluid shift comparable to that found in astronauts was indeed observed. Sonography has shown that the blood flows to the thorax and accumulates in the heart, provoking a dilation of the right auricle. The heart "interprets" this phenomenon as if it were a genuine increase in blood mass and therefore as a "flood" in the upper body. This false, yet understandable interpretation, sets off a whole series of neuroendocrine reactions designed to amplify the output of urine momentarily, with a resulting water loss and reduction in plasma volume (Figure 14).

These reactions are set in motion in the heart itself where the atrium wall contains areas rich in nerve endings from the pneumogastric nerve. These baroreceptors are sensitive to variations in blood volume. The redistribution of the blood mass stimulates them, and the resulting nerve impulses are sent to the nervous centres in the brain. Once informed, the nerve centres provoke an abrupt and significant decrease in vasopressin. O. R. Gauer and J. P. Henry had already observed this hormonal response in dogs after dilation of the right cardiac atrium using a small balloon. Aldosterone also decreases due to a reduction in renin secretion. In addition, it seems logical that atrial dilation must induce a sudden release of ANP.

The lower level of aldosterone associated with the reduction in vasopressin and the increase in ANP secretion induce a lower water absorption in the nephrons and, therefore, an increase in urinary excretion. Finally, excessive diuresis leads to water loss and consequently to hypovolemia, i.e., to a reduction in plasma volume.

This brief overview of the mechanism set in motion by blood redistribution is based on bed rest or water immersion experiments carried out in dogs or humans. This raises the question whether the same phenomenon, often described as the Henry-Gauer reflex, can also be observed in space. An exact answer is not possible, as the results of numerous investigations are often divergent and very different from ground simulation experimental findings:

- Hypertrophy of the cardiac cavities was observed on the first sonographies carried out in space on French astronaut Jean-Loup Chrétien. However, it is now known that this phenomenon in only temporary since the dilation of the left ventricle was seen only during the very first hours of flight. Indeed, if a decrease in leg volume is a sign of blood shift, there is nothing to indicate that all the redistributed blood mass ever reaches the thorax, the neck and the head. It is thought to be more likely that a portion of the blood is concentrated in the abdominal viscera. It should also be remembered that the puffy face observed in all astronauts is not due to a shift in blood but rather to interstitial fluid infiltrating the tissues, i.e., to extracellular fluid coming from other parts of the body.
- Hormonal reactions: a decrease in aldosterone secretion and a conversely exaggerated ANP synthesis have been observed in astronauts during space flights as well as ground-based simulations, as Gharib and A.I. Grigoriev have demonstrated. On the other hand, vasopressin measurements have given very different results. While a decrease in the blood vasopressin level has been repeatedly noted, studies carried out by Carol Leach on shuttle astronauts have shown an increase in hormone to a level of 360% at the very beginning of a flight.
- Increased diuresis: this phenomenon is constant during the early phase of ground-based experiments yet has never been observed in astronauts. However, the decrease in plasma volume, also characteristic of simulation experiments, is still observed in astronauts, proving again that nothing is simple.
- In addition, not all responses can be ascribed to microgravity. In particular, stress is common at the onset of missions and varies depending on the individual. Stress also disturbs the neuroendocrine system but is absent in ground-based simulation experiments.

TIME COURSE OF CARDIOVASCULAR RESPONSES

As mentioned above, the first minutes of flight cause the redistribution of blood and interstitial fluid that results in an entire series of neurohormonal reactions. All these phenomena are characteristic of an initial phase known as the adaptation phase. Later, around the third or fourth day, these disturbances slowly attenuate and the astronauts enter into a steady state or adapted phase: blood mass and interstitial fluid shifts cease, but the "puffy face" and "bird legs" phenomena continue. The astronauts can, of course, drink freely, yet diuresis, which can now be accurately measured, is often less than preflight levels.

- Regarding fluid regulation, the level of many hormones in the blood gradually returns to normal values. In contrast, ANP secretion is inhibited since the ANP blood level is down by 60% after a few days.

The hypovolemia that appears during the first few days does not increase: the plasma volume is 15 to 20% less than preflight values. Studies using radioactive oxygen have shown that this phenomenon is associated with a 3% decrease in body water content. As there is no increase in urinary output, this can be considered to be the result of a decreased water and food intake, no doubt because a spacecraft is not the best place for fine dining!

The persistent hypovolemia and lower water content are part and parcel of the weight loss observed in all astronauts, a phenomenon noted after the very first flights, although weight measurements had only been taken before and after the flight. A device using oscillatory springs has since been designed to replace conventional scales, which are obviously useless in weightlessness. This new device has shown that astronauts lose 2 to 3 kg after the first few days. Weight eventually stabilizes but can still decrease due to calcium loss and progressive muscular atrophy. A record loss of 5 kg was observed after seven days spent aboard the Mir station by an astronaut who did not suffer from motion sickness and had taken no medication. In addition, his diuresis and sodium loss (sodium normally retains water) had been reduced during the entire mission. It is clear that such individual variations do not make the physiologist's task any easier.

- Regarding the cardiovascular system itself, microgravity could disturb the heart and blood vascular system by inducing blood redistribution. In fact, many studies have demonstrated that the cardiovascular system can adapt to the space environment. Furthermore, as will be discussed later, some changes are not related to microgravity.

When studied using traditional methods, the heart does not seem to undergo serious modifications, although a slight tachycardia, or increase in heart rate, is frequently observed. Arterial pressure remains normal or may increase slightly at the beginning of a flight. In long-term flights it drops below normal values. Sono-cardiography is frequently used to measure heart volume. It has already been mentioned that the left ventricle volume increases slightly at the beginning of a flight, as does the amount of blood ejected with each contraction. Later on, the cardiac volume returns to baseline values. A post-flight reduction in the heart volume is observed, but individual variations are frequent.

More recently, another parameter, central venous pressure or CVP, i.e., the pressure of the blood entering the heart, has been studied. For many years it was believed that the blood shift to the thorax would increase CVP. On Earth, pressure is measured outside the right atrium in the superior vena cava, a large vessel that receives all the blood from the upper part of the body. In space, after several somewhat "indirect" measurements, the CVP was finally measured on three shuttle astronauts. Before launch, a narrow catheter was introduced in an arm vein up to the vena cava, very close to the right cardiac auricle. Everything went well, and the astronauts removed the catheters after 24 hours in space. Contrary to expectations, there was an increase in CVP but this response was quickly modified, and the measurements finally gave values only slightly inferior to preflight figures.

This surprising result might have led to the belief that Henry Gauer's hypothesis was no longer valid in the case of astronauts. In fact, it was quickly understood that these apparently paradoxical results were not due to microgravity, but to the astronaut's position prior to launch. During the final hours leading up to launch and the first hours of weightlessness, the astronauts are in a supine position with their legs up and bent at the knees. This position obviously causes a blood shift to the thorax and the heart and explains the slight temporary increase in CVP. Thus the blood and interstitial fluid shift occurs long before the astronauts are exposed to true weightlessness. Later on, the low CVP level and its persistence during the flight is proof that the heart has adapted to the absence of gravity.

The contractility of the myocardium or cardiac muscle is also of interest. The myocardium appears to be unaltered, as shown by the electrocardiograms performed on many astronauts. There is even an increase in the QRS wave amplitude, which corresponds to the ventricular contraction. However, a slight increase in the PR interval could indicate a small disturbance in the flow between the atria and the ventricles.

Other studies carried out by various scientists, and in particular P. Arbeille, have focused on local blood circulation. Both Doppler and sonography studies demonstrated increases in vascular resistance (calculated from systolic and diastolic flow) in the femoral artery, which irrigates the leg. An increase in the cerebral blood flow was also observed, rapidly followed by a stabilization at a normal or lower than normal value. The very low extent of these modifications is additional proof of the body's remarkable capacity to regulate cerebral blood flow. Concerning venous circulation, compliance or the capacity to be distended progressively increases up to the tenth day of flight and then tends to return to preflight levels.

The facts reported here show that the cardiovascular system, although operating under abnormal conditions, adapts to weightlessness in the majority of cases. Indeed, disturbances have seldom been reported. The most serious incident was an arythmia, which forced Alexander Laveikin to return prematurely to Earth after a five-month mission aboard the Mir station. The condition disappeared upon return to terrestrial gravity. Modifications of heart rate, which were not considered to be serious, also occurred in astronauts who walked on the moon. The same phenomena can occur during EVAs.

In spite of the small number of accidents and the noteworthy adaptation capacity of the human cardiovascular system to weightlessness, it is obvious that this system and the blood flow regulatory mechanism cannot be operating as they usually do. Indeed, in space, changing body position does not produce the vasoconstriction reflex that prevents the accumulation of blood in the lower parts of the body when changing to an upright position on Earth. The regulatory mechanisms of blood circulation are at rest in weightlessness. This is known as cardiovascular deconditioning.

The latter phenomenon and the persistence of a decreased plasma volume explain the appearance of minor problems upon returning to Earth when moving from a horizontal to an upright position. The astronaut is subject to dizziness, nausea, vomiting and fainting spells characteristic of a state of orthostatic intolerance (cf. Figure 13). These symptoms are only temporary and their seriousness can be reduced by the repeated use of a special device worn on the lower part of the body at the end of the flight. Creating a negative pressure for a few minutes causes a temporary return of the blood mass to the lower body, i.e., a blood distribution comparable to that observed under normal gravity. This technique, known as LBNP (low body negative pressure, Figure 15),

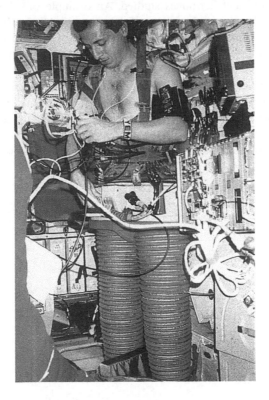

FIGURE 15 *Lower body negative pressure (LBNP)*

LBNP is a countermeasure to space deconditioning, and to the orthostatic intolerance that occurs just after a space flight. The astronaut wears trousers in which a vacuum is created. This induces a fluid shift, similar to the one that occurs on Earth when man goes from a lying to an upright position.

is nowadays combined with the intake of 1 liter of saline solution just prior to the return to Earth in order to cause water retention and thus restore a normal plasma volume. Thanks to these countermeasures and the physical exercises performed throughout the flight, the cardiovascular deconditioning does not last longer than between a few hours and 2 days on average and may not occur at all after landing. For long-term missions, the period of orthostatic intolerance may be longer. In the case of one Soviet cosmonaut it lasted 30 days after staying several months in space. A new, simple technique using a cuff or "bracelet" worn loosely on the thighs of the cosmonauts appears to be an efficient countermeasure since it stops the redistribution of the blood mass, thus decreasing the troubles it causes and even reducing the level of hypovolemia.

Despite the adaptation capacity of the cardiovascular system and the efficiency of certain countermeasures, there are still many unknowns, such as the frequent variation observed between ground-based and in-flight results. Furthermore, all the factors that might affect the responses of the cardiovascular system have not yet been studied, or at least insufficiently so, notably the hormone receptors in the organs sensitive to the different hormones studied. An example of7 this is urodilatin, a recently discovered hormone that plays a fundamental role in sodium excretion. On the other hand, it cannot be assumed that the heart would resist missions lasting several years in spite of the remarkable adaptive capacities it has already shown. Structural alterations to the myocardium and modifications in its metabolism were observed in rats after only two weeks of flight, highlighting the need to continue pursuing studies on Earth and in space for a better understanding of the reactions of the cardiovascular system to weightlessness. It is certain, however, that this research, indisputably stimulated by the development of astronautics, will lead to a better knowledge of the regulatory mechanisms of the cardiovascular system.

6 The Skeletal System and Weightlessness

The effects of weightlessness on the skeletal system constitute a serious problem in space medicine. The calcium loss to which astronauts are subject can lead to bone alterations thus making weightlessness a limiting factor or drawback in long-term missions. Weightlessness might induce a bone fragility that could harm an astronaut during long-term missions and even more so after returning to Earth. In addition, the absence of gravity can have repercussions on bone tissue related metabolism, i.e., calcium and phosphocalcium metabolism.

Calcium is one of the mineral elements that play an essential role in the human body: it is involved in functions as various as muscle and myocardium contraction, nervous impulse transmission, blood coagulation, cell permeability and hormone signalling to the cells. Maintaining the plasma calcium level or calcemia in the blood at its normal value of 100 mg/liter (or 5 mEq/1) is fundamental. However, the nutritional supply of calcium varies from day to day. Humoral regulatory mechanisms therefore come into play to increase or decrease calcium excretion through urine and feces accordingly. In addition, constant exchanges between bone and blood ensure that the plasma calcium balance is maintained.

In order to understand the changes in bone tissue occurring in space, a brief histological and physiological review will highlight once again the influence of gravity.

BONE DEVELOPMENT AND RESTRUCTURING

The human skeleton consists of long bones such as the tibia and the femur, short bones like those of the wrist or ankle, flat bones such as the skull and irregular bones like vertebrae. Gravity affects the long bones of the lower limbs and the vertebrae, which are considered antigravity bones since they support body weight in the upright position. At each extremity of the long bones is an expanded portion called epiphysis. The central section of the bone located between the epiphyses is a thin shaft called the diaphysis; the intermediary part between the two is the metaphysis.

The diaphysis is made up of compact bone tissue enclosed by the periosteum, which is a tough, fibrous membrane. The epiphysis and metaphysis are composed of spongy or cancellous bone tissue made of thin bars called trabeculae that are fused together and surround intercommunication spaces or medullary cavities. They contain the bone marrow that produces the blood platelets and a large number of blood cells, including red cells and granular leucocytes.

The compact bone tissue of the diaphysis is made up of small cylindrical structures known as osteons or haversian systems (Figure 16). Each one has a very

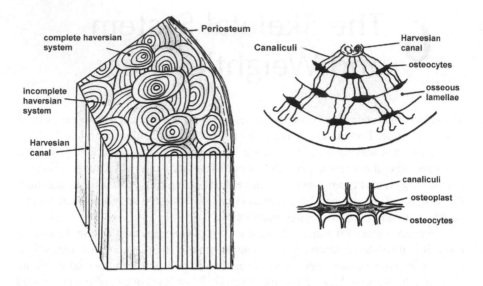

FIGURE 16 *Bone architecture*

Left: the diaphysis of a long bone consists in cylindrical parallel haversian canals or osteons. In a cross section, an haversian system appears to be made up of circumferential lamellae. Right: bone cells are located in small lacunae between lamellae and are connected to each other by canaliculi that branch out from a central canal.

narrow central canal called the haversian canal containing vessels and nerves. The wall of each osteon is made up of small cylinders; in a cross section; each osteon is seen to consist of several concentrically arranged lamellae (like an onion) that are about 10 microns thick.

The osteon lamellae are the essential components of bone tissue. Like all connective tissue, they contain an intercellular substance or bone matrix. In bone, the intercellular substance is highly calcified and contains large amounts of calcium carbonate and phosphate crystals in the form of apatites. Bone tissue contains up to 45% calcium, making the skeleton the largest reserve of calcium in the body: more than 95% of the 1250 g of total body calcium is stored there. Despite this high mineral content, bone would be fragile and poorly resistant if the bone matrix did not contain a network of small collagen fibers comparable to those found in other connective tissue like the dermis of the skin.

Bone tissue also contains cells called osteocytes, situated in small lacunae. Many thin canals, the bone canaliculi, arise from the lacunae and penetrate the bone matrix in all directions. The most internal canaliculi reach the central canal of the osteons. The osteocytes do not divide and appear to have a slow metabolism. Nutrients come from the blood capillaries of the central canal, penetrate in the canaliculi and reach the osteocytes. The canaliculi also allow calcium to be exchanged between bone and blood.

In the fetus and in children, bones have a different structure. In a first phase, the bone rudiment (or primordium) is made of cartilage wrapped in a connective envelope called perichondrium. Blood vessels penetrate the central part of the rudiment, and its disappearance gives rise to the primary medullary cavity. The perichondrium

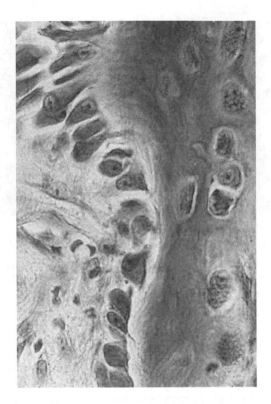

FIGURE 17 *Formation of bone tissue (see Color figure III at the end of the book)*

Young bone cells or osteoblasts secrete an interstitial substance. In a second step, calcium is deposited in it. Osteoblasts become osteocytes located in the lacunae, which are surrounded by a calcified interstitial substance. (Pr. M. Maillet, Fac. Med., Paris.)

then transforms itself into periosteum and produces a peripheral sheath of compact bone that constitutes the wall of the future shaft. At the same time, two epiphyseal cartilage plates appear between the cartilaginous epiphysis and the diaphysis, which mark off the medullary cavity at its two extremities. The epiphyseal plates form new cartilage and narrow bone bars that extend in the medullary cavity. These bars constitute the endochondral bone.

Osteoblasts, which give rise to endochondral and periostic bone, develop from undifferentiated stem cells situated in the perichondrium and the medullary cavities (Figure 17). The stem cells actively divide and give rise to new cells or osteoblasts that differentiate slowly. The osteoblasts have an important metabolic activity: they secrete the organic component of the bone matrix and the collagen fibrils embedded within it. Calcium and phosphate ions come from the blood and precipitate in the bone under the influence of an enzyme, alkaline phosphatase, which is secreted by the osteoblasts. When an osteoblast is surrounded by a calcified matrix, its activity stops and it becomes an osteocyte.

The primary periostic bone and the endochondral bone have a short life span and are progressively destroyed by large cells called osteoclasts (Figure 18). The

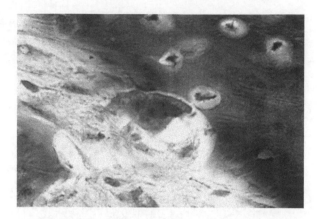

FIGURE 18 *Destruction of bone tissue (see Color figure IV at the end of the book)*

The destruction of bone tissue is associated with the presence of giant cells, osteoclasts, derived from cells in the marrow. They produce a substance that dissolves the bone, giving rise to a Howship's lacuna. This cycle of resorption and bone formation continues throughout life. (Pr. M. Maillet, Fac. Med., Paris.)

latter arise from the fusion of several blood monocytes. Osteoclasts settle on the surface of periostic bone or the trabeculae of endochondral bone. Bone is eroded and osteoclasts occupy little pits on the surface of the bone, called Howship's lacunae, which progressively increase in volume. Enzymes present in the osteoclasts are involved in bone resorption.

The opposite phenomenon, osteogenesis, immediately follows bone resorption and blood vessels and connective cells transformed into osteoblasts penetrate the lacunae. These cells attach themselves to their surface and give rise to a first lamella of bone. Shortly afterwards, new osteoblasts appear and position themselves on the first cylinder to form a second, smaller one. The lacunae gradually shrink and finally give rise to a haversian system made of several nested cylinders. Haversian bone tissue thus replaces the primary periostic bone.

Ossification might appear to be a simple process at first glance, but it is complicated by the fact that this primary haversian bone is subject to profound changes. Osteoclasts dig new lacunae, eating away some of the primary osteons. Secondary, tertiary osteons succeed each other in such a way that the adult bone is ultimately made of haversian systems. The osteons form the compact bone tissue in the diaphysis. The two epiphyses are also made of haversian bone but, in this case, the haversian bone is a spongy or cancellous tissue. The epiphyseal plates, which give rise to new cartilaginous tissue and new endochondral bone, finally disappear at the end of the growth period of adolescence.

These structural changes are not surprising since children's bones become longer and thicker without decreasing their mechanical properties. The diameter of the diaphysis, for instance, progressively increases. Resorption of primary tissue and formation of new bone occur simultaneously, and this bone remodelling will continue throughout the entire growth period.

It is easy to understand these phenomena in children but less so in adults. This process never actually stops so that when growth has obviously ceased, bones continue to be destroyed and replaced by new bone tissue in adults and even the elderly. Osteoblasts and osteoclasts are still present, notably in the cancellous bone of the metaphysis and epiphysis. These structural changes show that calcium is constantly being fixed and released by bone. This is precisely the origin of the calcium exchange between blood and bone described at the beginning of this chapter. It should be noted, however, that of the 6 g of calcium bound to or released from the skeleton each day, only 300 mg comes from this exchange. The remainder depends upon the mechanism of homeostatic regulation of calcemia. In this case, exchanges are still made between blood, bone matrix, and the interstitial fluid surrounding the osteocytes and circulating in the osteon canaliculi. There is no bone resorption, however, and these exchanges take place without the osteoclasts. This process is very rapid, and its increase results in a higher calcium excretion in the urine within a few hours; whereas, the consequences of increased bone remodeling only appears after several days or weeks.

If the cellular mechanism of bone resorption is understood, that of the second regulatory system of calcemia remains partly unknown. It is probable that the osteocytes play a role although how they are brought into play remains to be elucidated. They can be stimulated by electrical phenomena: indeed, and under the influence of movements and postural changes, certain bone parts undergo new constraints with the appearance of slight distortions. Experimental conditions have shown that a bending movement on a bone can cause variations in the electrical potential on the different sides of the bone. Electrical signals reaching the osteocyte membrane might cause calcium exchanges and even remodeling. The osteocytes, long considered simple cells in a state of rest, might intervene at any time in bone structure, as will be reported later. Space research has provided interesting results in this field and has given us a better understanding of the role played by gravity and osteocytes in the maintenance of bone structure.

THE ROLE OF HORMONES

Calcium exchanges between blood and bone, and remodeling in particular, are controlled by humoral, vitamin and hormonal factors:

- Vitamin C, so often used as an energizing factor, does not act directly on calcium but rather on the bone matrix. In the case of C avitaminosis, bone matrix formation is disturbed, and the calcification of new bone cannot take place normally.
- Vitamin D (or to be more precise 25-hydroxycholecalciferol) used to be given to children at one time in the form of cod-liver oil to stimulate growth. It does not act directly on bone but stimulates intestinal absorption of calcium and phosphates in the diet.
- The parathyroid, made up of four small glands hidden in the fibrous capsule of the thyroid gland, secretes parathyroid hormone or PTH. PTH stimulates bone resorption, and when administered in large quantities

causes the appearance of numerous osteoclasts and a rarefying of bone trabeculae while the urinary excretion of calcium increases. It also stimulates the intestinal absorption of calcium.

- Calcitonin has a curious origin. It is formed in the thyroid gland by C cells, which migrate over a long distance in the fetus. Whereas most thyroid cells come from an outgrowth of the digestive tract wall, C cells come from the ganglionic crest that represents the rudiments of the spinal ganglions in the nervous system.

PTH raises the blood calcium level while calcitonin has the opposite effect. Its mechanism of action is not well understood, but it appears to decrease bone resorption. Under experimental conditions, calcitonin induces a significant decrease in the number of osteoclasts as well as structural alterations providing evidence that there has been a slowing down in the functional activity of these cells.

Finally, other hormones act on bone tissue, or rather on osteogenesis. Growth hormone, which is secreted by the pituitary gland, acts on the epiphyseal plate in children, causing the bone to increase in length. Testosterone, the male sex hormone, stimulates protein synthesis and the formation of bone matrix. Some adrenal gland hormones such as the glycocorticoids (cortisone for instance) inhibit collagen synthesis and decrease the formation of bone tissue.

THE INFLUENCE OF GRAVITY

Many factors can affect bone tissue and calcium metabolism at any one time. However, the list of these factors would be incomplete without considering the influence of mechanical factors, which are of particular interest as they have allowed the effect of gravity on bone tissue to be understood.

As mentioned above, gravity creates weight and is therefore responsible for the pressure the body exerts on a large part of the skeleton. This results in a mechanical constraint on bones. Its influence on osteogenesis is obvious, as bone architecture is linked to the presence of mechanical constraints, compression force and tensile force (the resistance to lengthwise stress generated by muscle contraction). In the tibia shaft, for example, all haversian systems are parallel to the axis of the bone in order to offer the greatest mechanical resistance to the gravitational force. The same is true of the trabeculae of cancellous bones. Bed rest or immobilization in a cast clearly shows the influence of gravity. In all cases a decalcification as well as a decrease in bone mass are observed following an increase in bone resorption. In other words, the disappearance of mechanical constraints induces bone loss, i.e., more or less extensive osteoporosis.

In animals, various experiments have provided conclusive results. For example, when part of the ulna is removed from a sheep's hind leg, the pressure from body weight is exerted on the radius, another bone of the same limb. When this bone is submitted to new mechanical constraints, it develops, thickens and becomes more resistant. In another experiment, fixing a metal plate to the shaft of a bone is found to decrease the influence of gravity. The plate acts as a splint and puts the corresponding segment of the bone at rest, making it more or less subject to bone resorption, which results in the appearance of many osteoclasts. More recently, experiments have been carried out using the suspended rat technique. Because the rat rests only on its forelegs, there is no mechanical constraint on its hind legs. Histological examination of the hindquarter bones showed osteoporosis, or decalcification, and the appearance of numerous osteoclasts. These phenomena only affect the bones of the hind legs, which clearly demonstrates that the responses are due to the disappearance of the influence of gravity. Similar responses have been obtained with apes kept in a seated position for periods of up to six months; the spongy bone of the vertebrae became more rarefied than the compact shaft of the long bones. It is important to know that it took 40 months for the bones to recover their original resistance.

THE EFFECTS OF SPACE FLIGHTS

Many observations have confirmed that bone tissue is, despite its appearance, a living tissue. As such, it is prone to structural modifications caused by various factors, and it is now possible to understand the changes gravity induces in the skeleton and consequently on calcium metabolism. However, it appears that not all responses to space conditions have adverse effects on the skeleton. For instance, because of the absence of body weight, the compression load exerted upon the intervertebral discs disappears, hence making astronauts a few centimeters taller! However, back pain is often associated with this phenomenon, which disappears upon returning to Earth (Figure 19).

Now, it is clear that microgravity induces alterations in bone and calcium metabolism. Decalcification was observed in 12 of the astronauts on the Gemini and Apollo-7 and -8 flights in 1969. Studies in bone density using X-rays showed that bone calcium loss was on the order of 3.2%.

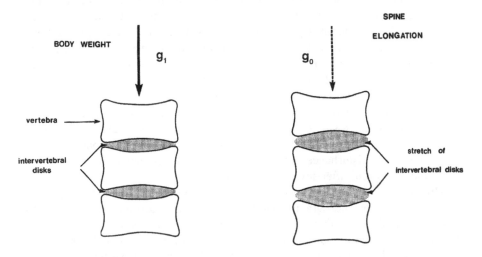

FIGURE 19 *The spine and weightlessness*

In space, the pressure on the spine disappears. The intervertebral disks become distended, making the astronauts a few centimeters taller.

Aboard Mir, research using more sophisticated techniques, like pre- and post-flight dual photonic densitometry, have shown a mean decrease of bone mineral density of about 0.3% per month in the cortical part of the tibia and up to 0.9% in cancellous bone. Decalcification only occurs in weight-bearing bones and not, for instance, in the radius. Demineralization is roughly correlated with mission duration but varies with each individual. Given the restricted number of astronauts in space missions, this variability could be an obstacle to statistical analysis of the results. Bone loss has also been observed during ground experiments, and these studies have shown that bone density can conversely increase in non-bearing bones like the skull.

The logical consequence of bone decalcification is the release of calcium and phosphate into the bloodstream. This phenomenon is nearly without consequence on calcemia, however, since regulatory phenomena immediately accelerate calcium excretion. A small amount is eliminated in the urine, and urinary calcium levels quickly increase before stabilizing around the 30th day of flight. A large amount of calcium is also eliminated in the feces, a phenomenon that increases with time. This eventually leads to daily calcium losses. For example, an average of 25 g of calcium per astronaut were lost after the 84-day flight of Skylab-4, which represents a significant amount given that the total human body calcium is just slightly over 1 kg. Calculations have shown that a 1-year mission would cause a loss of 300 g in the absence of countermeasures, which represents about a quarter of the body calcium content. An increase in the urinary excretion of hydroxyprolin is also observed but this is not surprising since this molecule is one of the components of bone collagen.

Confronted with these facts, questions are raised as to how bone loss occurs, how serious it is and how it can be slowed down. The origin of decalcification appears to be simple: microgravity puts part of the skeleton at rest and, under these conditions, bones are known to be subject to decalcification or osteoporosis. Microgravity might disturb the bone remodelling process by increasing bone resorption, decreasing osteogenesis, or both. Little is known since no systematic histological study has yet been undertaken during the different stages of a space flight. Although bone biopsies are routine in hospitals, they are difficult to perform in a space cabin, and in any case, the improvement of new imaging techniques should eventually replace such procedures. In addition, decalcification can result at least in part from a disturbance in calcium exchange between bone matrix and blood without inducing immediate changes in osteogenesis and resorption processes. In good agreement with this assumption, a slight increase in blood and urinary calcium has been noted within the first hours of a space flight. The precocity of these responses can only be explained by a disturbance in the regulatory system. An increase in bone resorption could only occur after several days or weeks.

Hormones regulating calcium and bone tissue metabolism could be responsible for bone loss under microgravity. Modifications seen in astronauts are difficult to interpret since they are often discrete and inconsistent. An early and brief increase in vitamin D level in the blood has been observed. An increase in calcitonin after a 7-day flight and a decrease after a several-month flight were also reported. The level of PTH in the blood of the astronauts of the Skylab and Spacelab missions was unchanged but doubled after Russian missions lasting 211 to 237 days. Changes in the levels of other hormones involved in calcium metabolism can occur: the level of cortisone, growth hormone and insulin in the blood tends to increase but this could be attributed to stress. Interpreting these results is clearly not an easy task and the true mechanism of human bone loss under microgravity therefore remains to be completely elucidated. Only animal experiments including histological studies will allow a better understanding of skeletal responses to microgravity.

ANIMAL EXPERIMENTS

Rats are easy to manipulate and have therefore been used predominantly in experiments although their skeleton continues to grow throughout their life. In spite of this difference with the human skeleton, a great deal of research has been carried out, beginning with Cosmos-605 and continuing on Russian biosatellites as well as aboard the Shuttle. In all cases space flights resulted in bone loss. Osteoporosis causes the trabeculae of the long bone shafts to narrow and rarefy in a similar fashion to what can be observed in human beings (Figure 20). As in man, these responses can be theoretically related to reduced osteogenesis or an increase in bone resorption.

The first hypothesis was confirmed when microscopic studies revealed that the number of osteoblasts had been greatly reduced. However, this decrease in osteoblast differentiation was not immediate since no modification was noted after a five-day flight. Along with a decrease in the number of osteoblasts, their secretion activity was lower than normal, and the level of osteocalcin, a bone matrix protein synthesized by these cells, was lower in the blood and bone tissue of rats flown aboard Spacelab.

The decrease in osteoblast number is related to a slowing down in the differentiation of stem cells that gradually turn into osteoblasts. This phenomenon was shown by histological studies and with cell cultures started from humerus and vertebrae bones of rats on the shuttle SLS2 flight.

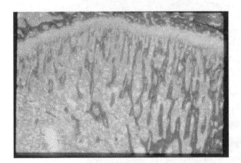 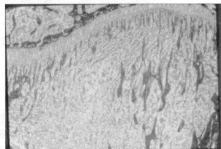

FIGURE 20 *Weightlessness and osteoporosis (see Color figure V at the end of the book)*

The figure shows the epiphyseal plates of a rat tibia. The cartilage cells multiply and, at the surface of cartilaginous bands, osteoblasts give rise to bone trabeculae (endochondral bone) separated by bone marrow. (From Vico, L. *et al.*)

Left: Controls.

Right: After a seven-day space mission (Biocosmos-1667). The space flight results in bone depletion or osteoporosis.

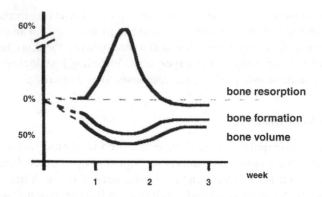

FIGURE 21 *The effect of weightlessness on bone*

In rat, exposure to weightlessness results in a temporary increase in bone resorption, lower bone formation and a resulting decrease in bone volume. (From Vico, L. *et al.*)

The higher bone resorption rate is also responsible for the observed decalcification. Thus, L. Vico found a definite increase in the number of osteoclasts in rats exposed to space flights for a period of 5 to 14 days (Figure 21). Such modifications in osteogenesis and bone resorption processes have also been observed in simulation experiments and, in particular, in experiments using the suspended rat technique. There again, the modifications were only noted on carrier bones.

In the experiments conducted in space and on the ground, the two mechanisms evolve as a function of time (Figure 22). The exaggeration of the resorption process

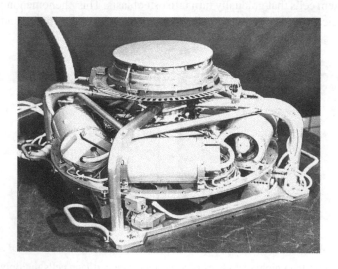

FIGURE 22 *An example of a 1 g centrifuge*

In space experiments, 1 g centrifuges are used aboard the spacecraft in order to compare biological objects exposed to microgravity or 1 g acceleration.

This centrifuge is a special device developed to study rats in space. (From Institute of Medical Problems, Moscow.)

is an ephemeral phenomenon, which appears earlier in simulation experiments than in experiments conducted under real weightlessness. On the other hand, the inhibition of osteogenesis persists at least for the entire length of the experiment, which varies between three and six weeks.

Thus two mechanisms can explain the appearance of decalcification after exposure to microgravity, whether real or simulated. Is bone growth also modified? The answer is no, at least concerning longitudinal growth. Indeed, E. Holton observed no significant difference in elongation, i.e., in lengthwise growth, in rats flown aboard the shuttle. On the other hand, exposure to weightlessness results in a reduced growth in width, which is ensured by the periosteum. This was demonstrated by several scientists using bone labeling before, during and after the flight. At each time, the fluorescent bone marker binds in areas where new bone is being elaborated. Markers produce colored rings, and the distance between two rings indicates the rate of growth. In this manner, it has been possible to show a reduction in osteogenesis at the periosteum level and, therefore, a growth reduction in terms of thickness.

In addition to experiments performed on adult bones, experiments conducted by J. J. W. A. Van Loon were also carried out on bones from the feet of mouse embryos cultivated *in vitro* on the IML-1 shuttle mission. The model system consisted in cartilage wrapped by perichondrium in which mineralization was starting. The bone continued to develop in a remarkable way, but studies using radioactive calcium and phosphate showed that mineralization was greatly reduced. Resorption by osteoclasts was enhanced.

Finally, it is to be emphasized that in spite of a certain degree of variability in the results—due to the often different experimental conditions—experiments carried out in space and on Earth clearly show that bone is sensitive to gravity. They have indeed led to a new model explaining the mechanism whereby gravity induces constraints on the skeleton.

A NEW MODEL

Under normal conditions on Earth, gravity and muscle contractions cause temporary bone deformities. These phenomena are weak yet cause a shift of interstitial fluid in the canaliculi and lacunae surrounding the osteocytes. The fluid movement stimulates the osteocyte membrane, and it is thought these cells produce chemical compounds that transform the stem cells into osteoblasts when they reach the medullary cavity. According to this model, proposed by several scientists and C. Alexandre (Saint-Etienne University) in particular, osteocytes could be considered to be mechanical receptors sending messages to the osteoblasts by mechanical transduction. Prostaglandins (a group of substances produced by the prostate and other organs) might be the signaling molecules responsible for transmitting this information.

While this model gives an important role to osteocytes, which have until recently been considered to be quiescent cells with little functional activity, it is also possible that gravity could affect stem cells and osteoblasts. Experiments carried out aboard the Russian biosatellite Bion-10 showed a delay in the differentiation of stem cells associated with morphological modifications. Furthermore when osteoblasts are cultivated on Earth on an elastic support, stretching the cultures affects the cells and causes an increase in protaglandin secretion. In the same way, osteocytes and osteo-blasts cultivated *in vitro* and submitted to the influence of fluid streams produce additional prostaglandin. This is an interesting result considering the role ascribed to fluid movement in the previously described model. It would seem, therefore, that osteocytes and osteoblasts are indirectly sensitive to the action of gravity. The hypothesis of a direct action can also be envisaged since osteoblasts placed onboard the Russian satellite Bio-10 proliferated less and underwent profound morphological changes even without any particular movement of their substratum.

RISKS AND COUNTERMEASURES

Bone changes in weightlessness are a serious problem. Indeed, even though coun-termeasures have reduced the seriousness of osteoporosis, it is estimated that bone loss still amounts to about a 0.5% loss per month.

Alterations in bone structure induce several risks for human beings on space missions. First of all, an elevated calcium mobilization might be followed by a precipitation of calcium outside bone tissue and, in particular, in the urinary tract where it can lead to the formation of renal stones. This could cause renal colic in space or after recovery, which requires quick treatment. Second, the osteoporosis that develops in weightlessness could result in lower bone resistance. Although this phenomenon does not appear to be serious for current missions, it might become a problem after a long-term mission when astronauts are reexposed to normal gravity after landing. Bone fragility might cause spontaneous fractures especially since bone loss seems to continue on Earth. Although there is a surprising degree of individual variation, it is clear that bone recovery is very slow and might last for a period equal to the space flight duration. The same time-course was observed in animals. One month after a space flight, the total trabecular bone volume in the tibia remained reduced. A third risk, the possibility of a fracture during a long-term mission, raises the problem whether repair processes are disturbed under microgravity. This idea has not escaped the attention of bone specialists who have studied the healing of a bilateral fracture surgically induced in rat fibula bones before takeoff aboard Cosmos-2044. Consolidation proved to be slower and the callous less resistant than normal. It remains to be known whether these results may be applied to astronauts.

In order to limit the effects of weightlessness, a number of measures have been thought of and applied, in particular for missions lasting several weeks or months.

The simplest method consists in giving the astronauts a calcium-rich diet. Indeed, simulation "bed rest" experiments on the ground where a subject is simply immo-bilized in bed have shown that the addition of calcium to the food intake delays the appearance of osteoporosis. Various drugs have also been tested. Ultimately, the preventive measure that might, *a priori*, be the most effective is physical exercise: pressure and traction create mechanical constraints on the skeleton, which should counter the effects of weightlessness. On long flights aboard Skylab, the shuttle, Russian space stations and the ISS, astronauts take up to two or three hours of exercise daily. Physical exercise is performed with the help of ergometric bicycles, travelators or extensors.

The results obtained with such countermeasures are only partly satisfactory because although the calcium loss is substantially attenuated, long missions are always associated with a loss in bone density and a negative calcium balance. When measuring the amount of ingested calcium as well as calcium eliminated in urine and fecal matter, it was found that, in spite of such daily exercises, the astronauts of Skylab had higher calcium excretion values than normal. Should one therefore change the nature and duration of physical exercise? We do not have the solution yet. Nevertheless, a simulation experiment on the ground convincingly suggests that the most efficient countermeasure should associate physical exercise with new medications. This experiment, conducted by Anatoly Grigoriev, Director of the Biomedical Problem Institute in Moscow, consisted of maintaining nine men under antihorthostatic hypokinesia for 360 days, a surprising length of time! The subjects received biphosphonate, a drug known to inhibit bone resorption, daily and by mouth. The men also did one to two hours of physical exercise per day. The results of this study are particularly interesting: the mobilization of bone calcium in the blood and the reduction in femoral neck bone density were greatly attenuated though not entirely abolished.

This demonstrates that the issue of what happens to bone in space is still far from being resolved. It is hoped, nevertheless, that new experiments will give further clues to reduce the effect of microgravity on the skeleton. New research avenues include the study of bone biopsies in man coupled with the administration of hormones on space flights as well as the use of new techniques such as computerized scanning.

CONCLUSION

In conclusion, space flights provoke serious bone modifications in man and animals. Although the role of weightlessness in this matter is now undisputed, the cellular and hormonal mechanisms involved as well as the preventive measures still raise many questions. It is safe to say, however, that space provides a particularly interesting means of studying the biology of bone tissue. This type of research opens new perspectives in medicine since the modifications observed under microgravity are very similar to those seen in osteoporosis, a condition that develops frequently in elderly subjects.

7 The Muscular System

Muscle is the second component of the locomotion system. As was found to be the case for bone, it is not surprising to discover that weightlessness induces alterations when the weight of the astronaut's body and surrounding objects disappears in the absence of gravity. Hence the amusing scene where an astronaut is performing a series of push-ups perfectly effortlessly! However, joke aside, the space environment results in such reduced activity that a space mission leads to significant changes in muscle mass and functional properties. As in the case of bone tissue, it seems useful to give a short overview of muscle structure and physiology in order to have a better understanding of the effects of microgravity on the muscle system.

MUSCLE FIBERS

Muscles are composed of large cells or fibers containing cylindrical thin elements known as myofibrils that are 1 to 2 μm in diameter (Figure 23). Myofibrils are the contractile element of the muscle fiber. Apart from the heart, there are two types of muscles in the human body:

1. Smooth muscle, present in the urinary and reproductive systems, in the digestive track and the walls of blood vessels
2. Skeletal muscle attached to bones by tendons

Cardiac and smooth muscle contractions are involuntary, whereas skeletal muscle contractions are voluntary.

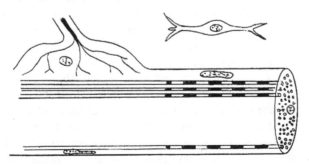

FIGURE 23 *Diagram of a striated muscle fiber*
The muscle fiber is a giant cell compared to a fibroblast. It contains many parallel myofibrils, which are the contractile element of the fiber.
The muscle fiber connects with nerve fibers in the motor end plate.

MUSCLE CONTRACTION

Skeletal muscle fibers are extraordinary: they are 4 to 5 cm in length and a few tenths of a millimeter in diameter. This is a far cry from usual cell size, which is generally 20 to 30 μm in length. Muscle fibers are highly differentiated and are therefore incapable of division. However, their structure is not stable. This is not surprising since it is well known that muscles develop with physical exercise. Muscle hypertrophy in this case is not due to an increase in the number of muscle fibers but to an increase in cell volume. Skeletal muscle atrophy from immobilization, for example, is of course the result of the opposite phenomenon. (It is worth noting, however, that very recent studies show that, in some cases, muscular fibers can be generated from stem cells.)

In addition to such temporary changes, muscle tissue is continually undergoing structural modifications with 1% of muscle proteins being renewed every day. This is an important metabolic phenomenon, since muscles represent 45% of a young adult's body weight. Because myosin and actin protein molecules, the components of myofibrils, are constantly degraded and synthesized, amino acids are always being released from muscle and replaced by new molecules.

The metabolic activity of muscle fiber can be modified: if the body receives a nonadequate nutritional supply or is subjected to prolonged immobilization, the breakdown process or catabolism increases and overtakes synthesis. The myofibrils are then fragmented and finally destroyed inside lysosomes, which are small vacuoles containing a battery of enzymes. Some hormones promote these phenomena, while others, like the male hormone testosterone, have the opposite effect. Insulin also plays an important role, as we shall see later.

THE EFFECTS OF GRAVITY

Thus muscle metabolism is regulated just as phosphocalcic metabolism, described in the previous section, is itself regulated. As with bone tissue, normal regulation of muscle metabolism supposes that the organism is living in a normal environment under the influence of gravity. Indeed, the role of gravity explains why muscles are made up of two kinds of fibers the structure and function of which are adapted to gravity. Type I fibers, or red fibers, are the larger of the two. They are rich in myoglobin, a red pigment similar to hemoglobin in red blood cells. They also contain numerous mitochondria, which are small organelles found in all cells. Mitochondria are enzyme-rich and constitute a source of energy for red fibers as they can break down certain compounds like fatty acids thanks to the oxygen bound by myoglobin. Type II white fibers contain less myoglobin and fewer mitochondria. The energy needed for their contraction comes from breaking down glycogen, a large molecule that belongs to the group of polysaccharides and is essentially composed of glucose molecules. Type I fibers have an oxidative-type metabolism while the type II fibers have a glycolytic-type metabolism.

The two types of fibers are distributed throughout the body in different ways. In certain animals, such as birds, some muscles only have one kind of fiber, making it possible to distinguish white muscles from red muscles. White and red muscles are physiologically very different. White muscles undergo short and rapid contractions—hence the name fast twitch fibers—which quickly lead to fatigue. Red muscles are capable of slow, sustained contractions—hence the name slow twitch fibers—allowing for greater stamina. In humans, the two types of fibers are found in every muscle though in variable proportions. The extensor muscles of the limbs and the paravertebral muscles, for instance, are muscles where red fibers are predominant. These posture muscles allow the body to remain upright and preserve its balance when moving. They are antigravity muscles without which the body would tilt forward and progressively bend over. It is therefore not surprising to learn that these muscles are affected by weightlessness.

THE EFFECTS OF WEIGHTLESSNESS

Anthropometric measurements made on different parts of the body have revealed alterations in the muscles of astronauts. These measurements were performed on Skylab and shuttle missions as well as on Salyut and Mir. A decrease in lower limb and especially calf volume was detected in every case after a few weeks in space. The results showed individual variation but could reach a value of 10%. Blood and interstitial fluid shift is one possible explanation, but this phenomenon alone cannot explain the modifications in leg volume since muscle atrophy has been detected by techniques such as magnetic resonance. Muscle atrophy appears rapidly, usually after between 8 and 11 days of flight, but can appear as early as the fifth day, as observed in one astronaut. Furthermore, the influence of gravity depends on the muscle, the volume decreasing by 3.9% in the calf and 6% in the quadriceps muscle of the thigh.

Functional modifications are associated with these structural variations, and it is logical for muscle power to be reduced after a space flight. For instance, after a 53-day mission aboard Skylab-3, leg muscle power decreased by approximately 20%. The decrease in arm muscle power is usually less pronounced since arm muscles do not struggle against gravity as frequently as leg muscles do on Earth. In addition, moving weightless objects requires less effort than on the ground. Experiments were also carried out in rats. After a seven-day mission, the muscles of rats on the flight were more subject to fatigue than the muscles of control rats.

Gravity-induced changes can also be demonstrated by electromyogram recordings, which measure muscle electrical activity. Muscle contractions are associated with a brief depolarization or action potential detected by placing electrodes on the muscle surface. The greater the muscle contraction, the higher the number of contracting muscle fibers and level of the corresponding electrical response. The results of studies performed after recovery show once again that muscles have undergone alterations and exhibit a decrease in contractility associated with a lower resistance to fatigue.

Regardless of the parameters studied, it is obvious that the muscle response is linked to the disappearance of mechanical constraints and to decreased muscular activity. The latter is induced by microgravity as well as hypokinesia due to limited movement inside the spacecraft. The same responses are also found in bed rest and animal experiments. For example, the volume of the rat soleus muscle in the posterior

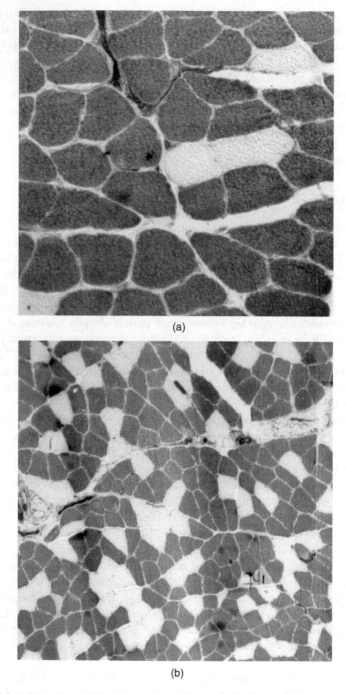

(a)

(b)

FIGURE 24 *Effects of weightlessness in the skeletal muscle structure (leg muscle)*

a: Rat control. Type I or slow twitch fibers (black) and type II or fast twitch fibers (white).
b: After a 7-day space flight, decrease in fiber volume and increase in the percentage of type
II fibers. (From Desplanches, D. *et al.*, 1990.)

part of the leg decreased by 25% after four days and 36% after seven days aboard the shuttle. Finally, exposure to microgravity clearly induces significant structural and functional modifications in skeletal muscle, which are easily measured using standard techniques. In addition, the changes are more pronounced because the microscopic structure of muscles is also significantly affected.

The first observations were carried out in 1985 on rats in Skylab-3 aboard Challenger. The effects of microgravity were surprising (Figure 24). Microscopic examination revealed that the muscles had undergone significant structural modifications: the diameter of all the muscle fibers decreased and the proportion of white fibers increased. Type I red fibers used for sustained effort and posture were replaced by type II white fibers. Furthermore, the space flight induced a decrease in the total mass of muscle proteins and changes in metabolism, which was converted to the glycolytic type characteristic of white fibers. Histological studies were not conducted on human beings until 1995 when pre- and postflight biopsies were performed on muscles from three then five astronauts during 5- and 11-day missions aboard the shuttle. This study was a remarkable example of international cooperation since American, Canadian, Danish and Japanese scientists took part in the experiment. The results demonstrated the adaptation capacity of human muscle to weightlessness. Muscle fiber diameter decreased by 15% to 30%, and the number of blood capillaries around the muscle fibers was down compared to preflight levels. The proportion of different fibers also changed, with type I fibers changing from a preflight level of 43% to 37% after the 5-day flight and type II fibers changing from 57% to 63%. After the 11-day flight, the proportion of type I fibers went from 45% to 39% and type II fibers from 55% to 61%. These results are in good agreement with those reported in animal experiments.

The question is now raised as to whether the structural and functional changes are induced by a decrease in protein synthesis, an increase in the breakdown process or a combination of both. Complementary studies confirmed the third hypothesis.

Indeed, in suspended rat experiments, the rate of protein synthesis in the soleus muscle decreased by 21% after the third day and even more on subsequent days. Molecular biology studies have shown that different steps of protein synthesis are affected. An increase in protein breakdown appears at a later stage. This is demonstrated by an increase in the activity of proteases, i.e., enzymes that degrade proteins. Complementary investigations suggest that gravity can affect genes regulating the synthesis of these enzymes. This result is of great interest although the weightlessness-induced signal that causes the inhibition of these genes remains obscure.

Biochemical investigations were also carried out in man. The results clearly show a higher level of muscle protein degradation. Indeed, the urine of astronauts contains many amino acids originating from muscle proteins as well as an elevated level of the muscle protein, creatinine. Although an astronaut's diet is protein-rich, the degradation of muscle proteins is such that nitrogen losses outweigh the gains and the nitrogen balance becomes negative.

Although metabolic changes partially explain the muscle atrophy observed in weightlessness, it is possible that other factors like the nervous system and hormones might be involved in the observed muscle responses.

Each muscle fiber is connected with a nerve fiber bound to a small raised area of the muscle cell surface known as the motor plate or neuromuscular junction. Each nervous impulse crosses the motor plate and causes the myofibrils to contract. Innervation is thus necessary for the striated muscle fiber to contract. However the role of the nervous system is not limited to this function alone, as cutting the motor nerve not only causes paralysis but also muscle atrophy. Although no paralytic phenomenon appears in weightlessness, electronic microscope studies carried out on rats after a biosatellite flight uncovered structural changes in the motor plates.

Hormones can also affect muscle tissue. On Earth, insulin activates the intake of amino acids and stimulates muscle protein synthesis. On this basis, it might be assumed that the increased degradation of muscle protein in microgravity could be related to a decrease in insulin secretion. In fact, measurements of insulin and glycemia (insulin decreases glycemia) did not give reproducible and therefore significant results. Furthermore, changes in insulin levels must be interpreted with care. Responses to hormones in general depend not only on their level in the blood but also on receptors located on target cells, i.e., the cells sensitive to a given hormone. The minor elevation in the glucose level and the threefold increase in insulin reported after shuttle flights could be due to an altered sensitivity to insulin due to changes in its receptors, as the American physiologist C. Leach suggested.

CONCLUSION

Muscles as well as bones are affected by exposure to microgravity and adapt to the absence of gravity through structural changes. However, the mechanisms underlying this adaptive capacity and the changes involved are still elusive. It is in part difficult to improve our knowledge of the effects of weightlessness precisely because of the daily exercise schedules imposed on astronauts to prevent skeletal muscle alteration and bone loss. Physical exercise has beneficial effects on the muscle system as it significantly decreases muscle atrophy and muscle protein breakdown. However, the results are not completely satisfactory, especially for long-term flights. For instance, after 366 days on Mir, and despite daily exercises, the strength of the leg extensor muscles decreased by approximately 50%. It should be added that large individual variations exist. It is obvious that astronauts do not all have the same physical condition before the flight or the same type of work to do during the space mission. It is worth noting that it can take several days or weeks for the functional capacities of the muscle system to become normal again. Improved exercises associated with the intake of certain drugs should be developed in the future in order to prevent microgravity-induced effects, especially in long-term missions.

8 The Vestibular Apparatus and Balance System

The third organ disturbed under weightlessness is the vestibular apparatus. Although it plays an essential role in everyday life, few people are aware of its existence. This is easily explained: whereas human beings are continuously made conscious of the world around them through sight, hearing, olfaction and touch detectors, the vestibular apparatus is an automatic system, sending subconscious information to the brain. Only pathological manifestations, for instance vertigo or motion sickness caused by a rocking ship, remind us of its presence.

The vestibular apparatus has a complex role to play. It is a part of the sensory motor system that controls body orientation, locomotion, accurate movement and eye motion. This control requires information coming not only from the vestibular system, but also from vision and proprioception (Figure 25). While vision can be considered to be independent from gravity, proprioception and, to a greater extent, the vestibular apparatus are affected by gravity. This explains why astronauts, as we shall see later, not only experience sickness but also many types of other disturbances.

PROPRIOCEPTION

Proprioception is the function that allows the brain to receive information from muscles, tendons and joints. Touch receptors located near the skin surface also participate in proprioception and body balance. That is the case for receptors located in the sole of the foot. In an upright position, body weight exerts a pressure on this area, thus stimulating nerve endings and subconsciously informing the brain that the body is upright. In the same way, nerve fibers in the region of the buttocks confirm that the body is seated.

Proprioceptive signals are also received from tendons, joints and muscles. The tendons contain Golgi corpuscles, which are small organelles, a few tenths of a millimeter in length, connected to nerve fiber endings. The Golgi corpuscles are stimulated when a muscle contraction induces the stretching of tendons. In addition, the fibrous capsules of joints contain small receptors. They are more or less compressed depending on the limb position and provide information relating to posture. Muscles also give proprioceptive information, which comes from small structures called neuromuscular spindles located between muscle fibers. Like muscle fibers, spindle fibers contain myofibrils capable of contraction. Each spindle is supplied with motor and sensory nerve fibers. When at rest the muscles are always slightly stretched, as are the spindles, which causes the departure of a few impulses toward nerve centers. If a muscle is contracted, the stretching of the spindles and the nerve

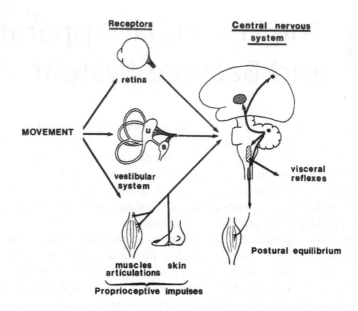

FIGURE 25 *Sensory and balance system on Earth*

On Earth, the central nervous system receives signals from vision, the vestibular apparatus and proprioception (nerve endings in muscles, tendons, joints and skin). These signals are responsible for body orientation and equilibrium.

impulse frequency decrease. The opposite occurs if the muscle is stretched by the contraction of opposing muscles. Finally, thanks to proprioception, nerve centers receive subconscious signals about muscle tension and position in different parts of the body.

THE VESTIBULAR SYSTEM

The vestibular system plays an essential role in balance. It is a part of the inner ear, which is located in the petrous part of the temporal bone at the base of the skull. The inner ear or labyrinth consists of a spiral canal called the cochlea, which is the seat of hearing, and the vestibular apparatus right beside it (Figure 26).

The vestibular apparatus consists of three semi-circular canals (SCCs) positioned at right angles to one another in three dimension. The SCCs are filled with a fluid or endolymph that moves when the head rotates; the stimulated canal is the one located in the plane of movement. In medicine, a simple way of examining these canals is to place the patient in a rotating chair and study his posture and eye movements. In space, the absence of gravity does not affect the function of the SCCs because gravity does not act at this level. On the other hand, the acceleration created by body movement does, both on Earth and in a spacecraft.

The vestibular apparatus also consists of two large sacs, the utricle and the saccule, which communicate with each other as well as with the SCCs. The utricle and the saccule are very sensitive to gravity, and their activity is consequently greatly

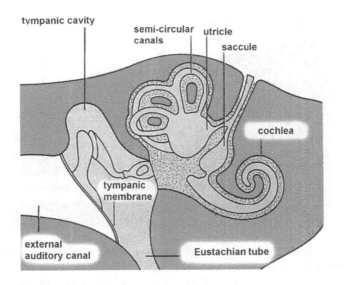

FIGURE 26 *Diagram of the ear*

The ear consists of three main parts (an internal, middle and inner part).
The inner ear comprises the cochlea and the vestibular system, which are responsible for hearing and equilibrium, respectively. The vestibular system consists of three semi-circular canals, which respond to rotation of the head, and two large sacs, the utricle and the saccule also called the otolith apparatus. The otolith apparatus is disturbed under microgravity.

disturbed in space, much to the astronauts' dismay. As with most hollow organs, the utricle and the saccule are covered by epithelium, which is a layer of closely packed cells (Figure 27). When viewed under a microscope, the epithelium appears to be composed of two kinds of cells: simple columnar cells known as supporting cells interspersed with round-shaped sensory cells which possess thin processes on their upper surface. The otolithic membrane, a thick gelatinous substance, covers the epithelium. Its lower face is hollowed out with small lodges into which sensory cell hairs penetrate. The upper face of the otolithic membrane is covered with small calcium carbonate crystals 10 micrometers in length (a micrometer being a thousandth of a millimeter) with a specific gravity of about 3. They are called otoliths or otoconia, which is why the utricle and the saccule are often referred to as the otolith apparatus. In addition, the lateral and basal faces of hair cells are surrounded by many nerve fibers. These are the endings of the vestibular nerve, the part of the auditory nerve that connects with the central nervous system.

The saccule and the utricle do not have the same orientation. When the body is upright, the epithelium is situated vertically in the saccule and horizontally in the utricle. If the saccule were to be examined directly, the otoliths and the otolithic membrane would be seen to slide in the direction of gravity because of their weight, causing the hairs to bend (Figure 28). By modifying the electrical properties of the cell membrane, this movement stimulates the nerve endings of the vestibular nerve,

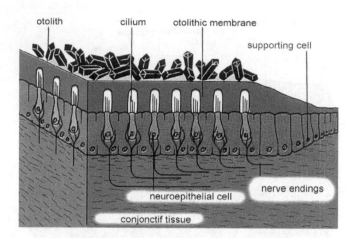

FIGURE 27 *Diagram of the macula structure in the utricle and saccule (maculae are thickened portions of utricle and saccule walls)*

The inner surface of the utricle and saccule maculae is lined with an epithelium that consists of supporting cells and ciliated or sensory cells. The cilia penetrate in a gelatinous membrane, the otolith membrane. Beyond this membrane are found small crystalline bodies known as otoconia or otoliths. The basal part of the ciliated cells is surrounded by nerve endings.

giving rise to a continuous flow of nerve impulses to the brain. This constitutes the basic activity of the otolithic apparatus. Meanwhile, the epithelium of the utricle is in a horizontal position so that the otoliths and otolithic membrane are not displaced. The hair cells of the utricle are at rest and do not send any impulses to the nervous centers.

When the head is tilted, the otoliths slide like any object with a weight in the direction of gravity, causing the hairs to bend and nerve impulses to be discharged.

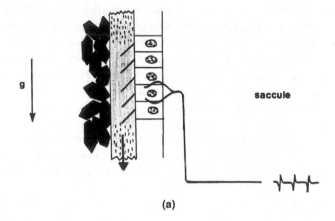

(a)

FIGURE 28 *Physiology of the otolith apparatus*

a) On Earth, in the upright position, the saccule epithelium is in the vertical position. Due to their weight, the otoliths tend to go downward and bend the cilia. Ciliated cells are stimulated and a signal is sent to the brain. In space, the otoliths of the saccule do not move and the brain receives no signals.

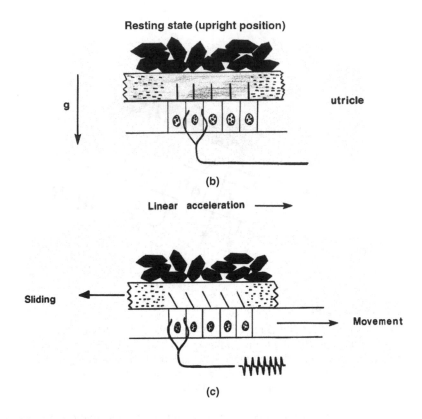

Resting state (upright position)

utricle

g

(b)

Linear acceleration ⟶

Sliding ⟵

Movement ⟶

(c)

FIGURE 28 (Continued)

b) On Earth, in the upright position, the epithelium of the utricle is in the horizontal position. As in space, no signal is sent to the brain in the absence of movement.

c) In space, when the astronaut moves in the spacecraft, the linear acceleration results in a displacement of the otoliths in the opposite direction. The bending of cilia stimulates the ciliated cells on Earth or under microgravity. The brain receives signals in both cases.

The degree of the response depends on the degree of head tilt. In this case, gravity acts as a reference vector, and it is thanks to this "plumb-line" that the otolithic apparatus informs the nervous centers to provoke the muscular responses necessary to maintain body equilibrium. The otolithic apparatus is also stimulated by linear acceleration, for instance, when walking faster or slower. Just like an object on a plate that is suddenly moved to one side, the otoliths and the otolithic membrane move in the opposite direction to the body and thus head movement. This tangential movement causes the hairs to bend again with the release of nervous impulses on Earth and in space.

These phenomena show that the brain constantly receives a great deal of information from vision, the proprioceptive system and the vestibular apparatus. This information is treated in a computer-like manner according to innate programs as well as acquired ones, as can be seen in young children gradually acquiring the reflexes that ensure their balance when they learn to walk. After following a highly complicated path through the spinal bulb, the cerebellum, the brain and the medulla, this information produces the motor responses that trigger muscular activity. It

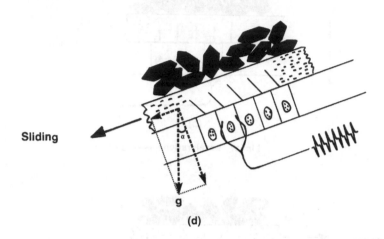

(d)

FIGURE 28 (Continued)

d) On Earth, when the head is tilted to one side, the otoliths slide down and the greater the roll, the greater the signal to the brain. In this case, gravity is a reference vector, and the signal depends on the angle between the vertical and the horizontal relative to the otolith membrane. In space, the otoliths do not move and ciliated cells are not stimulated. (From Planel, *H. L' Espace et la Vie.* Larousse, Paris, 1988.)

should also be noted that the three mentioned sources of information are linked to each other, this being especially true for vision and the vestibular apparatus. Indeed, the vestibular nucleus, situated in the spinal bulb, is linked both to the otolithic apparatus and the oculomotor nuclei, which are situated higher in the cerebral trunk and control eye movement. Oculovestibular interactions are in fact highly complex, though it is quite easy to be made aware of them. When the head rotates, it is obvious that the objects we are looking at remain motionless in our visual field. This is explained by the fact that the information from the vestibular apparatus, in this case the semicircular canals stimulated by the movement of the head, and the oculomotor nuclei order eye muscles to move the eyeballs in the opposite direction to the head movement. This constitutes the vestibulo-ocular reflex or VOR, created by signals from the visual and vestibular systems.

THE EFFECTS OF WEIGHTLESSNESS

Because posture and movement coordination bring into play very complex mechanisms in which gravity plays a role, it is not surprising that many disturbances occur during space flights. Due to the disappearance of body weight, the nerve endings in the sole of the foot and in the buttocks are no longer stimulated when an astronaut is standing or sitting. In the muscles, neuromuscular spindles continue to be somewhat stimulated according to muscle length, but this will not be so for tendon receptors, since muscular contractions are often weaker in weightlessness than on

Earth. Weightlessness also acts indirectly on the leg muscle receptors that normally participate in maintaining balance and are at rest in the case of astronauts.

The absence of gravity also disturbs vestibular activity. To begin with, there is nothing to cause the otoliths and their supporting membrane to slide downwards, as happens in the saccule when the body is in a vertical position or when the head is tilted sideways. Therefore, at this level, there is no information to convey. However, the sudden movements made by astronauts create linear accelerations that continue to stimulate the vestibular system. The mass of the otoliths does not disappear in weightlessness and thus otoliths continue to slide as they do on Earth.

In summary a significant amount of information provided by the otolithic system and by proprioception disappear in weightlessness thereby causing the brain to receive different information. Under these conditions, the majority of signals comes from vision and semi-circular canals, which remain unmodified. In weightlessness, the information supplied to the brain does not conform to the usual programs, thereby creating sensory conflict. This situation explains why space crewmembers experience so many disturbances:

- Illusions, which can lead to the impression that the body is floating or swaying, notably after sudden head movements, have been reported, as has the impression that the cabin walls and the equipment are moving when the astronaut is stationary. All these phenomena are explained by the close connection between the vestibular and oculomotor nuclei situated in the central nervous system. Weightlessness can also alter the illusions caused by certain conditions on Earth:
  - The sensation of movement when remaining stationary as a result of observing moving objects, similarly to what typically happens on a train. This sensation has been recreated by fixing optical equipment to the astronauts' head and projecting rotating visual scenes before their eyes. L.R. Young noted that such illusions increased during studies carried out aboard Skylab.
  - Illusions of proprioceptive origin are also elicited by mechanical vibrations applied to the tendons of the ankle in a stationary subject. This technique stimulates the proprioception receptors in the leg tendons and muscles, causing the sensation that the body is swaying to-and-fro. Research carried out during the Franco-Russian Aragatz, Antares and Altaïr missions aboard the Mir station demonstrated that these responses persisted in weightlessness, although they were greatly reduced. The same technique can sometimes cause actual swaying movements of the body but to a lesser degree than on Earth. Thus muscle proprioception does not disappear in microgravity but is merely modified. It is interesting to note that these modifications increase with the duration of the mission, but if the effects of gravity on muscles are reproduced using elastic bands, the responses to mechanical vibration return to normal during the first days of the flight.
  - Strange phenomena regarding posture also occur at the beginning of a mission. In the upright position on Earth, the body always tilts forward

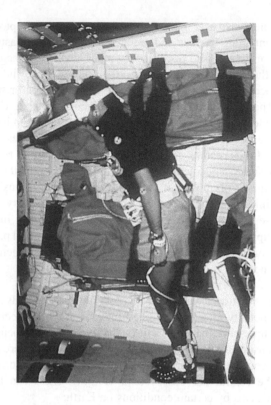

FIGURE 29 *Posture changes in space*
Under microgravity, the astronaut was asked to be in an "upright" position, with his body perpendicular to the spacecraft floor. With his eyes closed, thus in absence of vision, the astronaut could not judge his postural position and leaned forward.

by 1 or 2 degrees. However, when an astronaut is asked to stand upright, i.e., perpendicular to the floor of the spacecraft, his body tilts forward by 5, 10 and sometimes even 30 degrees, which would cause one to fall over on Earth (Figure 29).

• Finally, space motion sickness or SMS is the most clinically significant manifestation of neurosensory disturbances. As in terrestrial motion sickness, the symptoms of SMS are headaches and nausea that can lead to vomiting. More than 50% of all astronauts experience it even though all of them undergo very careful selection after being subjected to numerous vestibular tests. SMS is thus unpredictable. The astronauts' movements further increase the incidence of space motion sickness. It was generally absent during the first space flights when the volume of the capsule was very small and the astronauts had no choice but to remain seated. The volume of the Mercury cabin, for example, was only 1.3 m^3, while that of the Salyut craft was 100 m^3.

Typically, the first symptoms appear during the first hours of flight and resolve between 30 and 40 hours. However, a Russian cosmonaut experienced motion sickness after several months spent in space! The usual time course of SMS explains why it might hamper the work schedule on short missions. During reentry or just after landing, astronauts can also experience motion sickness.

Little is known about the mechanism causing SMS. We do know that body and, in particular, head movements are necessary to induce SMS. It is likely that the previously mentioned conflict between the sensory signals reaching the nervous centers might give rise to a dysfunction of the autonomous nervous system, thereby inducing a state of stress. Nervous centers such as the vomiting center are connected to the vagus nerve, which innervates the digestive tract and the stomach. This would explain the feeling of nausea and the vomiting reflex.

Pharmacology treatment is currently the method of choice for preventing or at least controlling SMS. More or less effective drugs, such as scopolamine can be used. Promethazine is administered either orally, as a suppository, or by intramuscular injection. It is so efficient that shuttle astronauts keep in their spacesuits the necessary equipment to inject themselves when the first symptoms of space motion sickness appear. Other methods are being studied, and notably the use of antagonists of the antidiuretic hormone, vasopressin. The rationale behind this is that secretion of this hormone might be involved since it is greatly increased when SMS occurs.

ADAPTATION AND PLASTICITY OF NERVE CENTERS

The temporary nature of SMS demonstrates that the neurosensory system adapts remarkably well to weightlessness. The "posture" experiment designed by A. Berthoz and F. Lestienne, which consisted of recording the electrical activity of an astronaut's leg muscles during a voluntary forward arm movement, confirmed this adaptability. Their research showed first of all that weightlessness reverses the muscle tone activity of the flexor and extensor leg muscles. At rest on Earth, extensor muscles play a prominent role in stopping the body from falling forward. However, the opposite occurs in space, leading astronauts to develop the new posture we have already mentioned. In space, astronauts develop a new strategy of movement as shown by simple actions such as picking up objects from the floor. Video cameras have filmed the movement of marks made at different points on the body and demonstrated that the bending of the legs and trunk is different in space and on Earth.

A great deal of research has also been conducted on vision. Eyesight, as we shall see later on, is not modified. On the other hand, weightlessness gives rise to alterations in eye movement. As already mentioned, when the head moves in one direction, the eyes move in the opposite direction; the vestibular system is involved in these compensatory eye movements, referred to as the vestibulo-ocular reflex (VOR). Although the activity of the vestibular apparatus is modified in weightlessness, the VOR persists and allows astronauts to have a normal vision of their environment. It is, however, possible to detect certain modifications, particularly when studying nystagmus. By this term, we designate a succession of slow and rapid eye movements that appear after a person has been rotated on a swivel chair. In medicine, the study of nystagmus is often used on patients suffering from dizziness. Nystagmus can also be induced when a device that displays moving scenery is placed on an astronaut's head. The results show that microgravity modifies nystagmus without hampering vision. Once again the nerve centers adapt.

In summary, it is clear that the disappearance of gravity, which is both a static force and a reference vector, greatly disturbs the nerve centers that control posture and movement coordination. These functional disturbances certainly reflect structural changes comparable to those found in animals after they have been removed from a labyrinth: loss of synaptic contacts (a place of contact between two nerve cells) followed by the appearance of new synaptic contacts. This ability to adapt requires the formation of new networks. On the other hand, morphological changes can occur in peripheral receptors: in the utricle and the saccule, the number of nerve endings around the hair cells increase. According to M. Ross, the vestibular receptors could thus compensate for the weightlessness of otoliths.

This neuronal plasticity in the balance apparatus allows astronauts to readapt to gravity after landing. For a few hours or sometimes a few days, astronauts experience minor problems related to microgravity-induced restructuring of nerve centers. When walking, they often have the sensation that their body is falling forward. They also experience orientation difficulties, veering to the left or right instead of walking in a straight line. The information coming from the two utricles is probably not identical on both sides. Movements requiring good coordination are often imprecise, as demonstrated by the example of Jean-Loup Chrétien who had to wait 24 hours before playing tennis normally again. Temporary problems also occur when the subject is stationary, and often a simple tilt of the head can lead to loss of balance and even falling. Such problems are usually significantly more pronounced after long-term flights, although individual variations can be substantial. Valeri Poliakov, for example, was able to stand up and walk without difficulty only a few hours after completing a 437-day mission aboard the Mir station.

THE IMPORTANCE OF COGNITIVE PHENOMENA

For a long time, research was concentrated on the influence of gravity and microgravity on relatively simple mechanisms such as those responsible for posture or vestibulo-ocular reflexes. It is now time to know if gravity also acts upon more complex processes such as body representation in space and the perception of one's orientation. Both of these phenomena rely on the complex mechanism of cognition, which requires the use of memory and the intervention of the brain.

In order to address this question, numerous neurobiological experiments were conducted aboard Mir and the space shuttle and, in particular during the Neurolab mission in April 1998 on the Columbia shuttle. Only the more striking results will be reported here and summarized very briefly:

- The first example concerns the effect of gravity on the phenomenon of mental rotation. Mental rotation occurs when two identical differently orientated objects are displayed. To compare them and confirm their identity, the brain imagines that they are parallel and must rotate them mentally to do so. The response rate depends on the size of the angle separating the two objects. In space, this response is more rapid, at least when objects are rotated about a roll or pitch axis. The astronaut's brain no longer needs to take gravity into account and has therefore one less factor to consider; hence, the more rapid response. This might explain the strange phenomenon frequently observed during many space missions: after several days, astronauts can read documents floating freely in the cabin, even when they are tilted at a 90-degree or greater angle in relation to the axis of their body. In space, the concept of being vertical is no longer relevant and, as the brain slowly adapts to this strange environment, mental rotation is easier to perform.

- When a human being moves, he is kept aware of the path he has traveled and is consequently able to know his spatial position. The messages gathered from different sensing receptors are then integrated in a particular structure known as the hippocampus, which is located in the brain. Studies conducted on the ground using rats have shown that as the rat moves along, the neurones of the hippocampus are stimulated, thus providing information about the path already traveled. Does gravity exert an influence in this case? B. MacNaughton provided the answer during the Neurolab mission by recording the neuronal activity of the hippocampus. This author showed that a cognitive map of the environment still appeared under microgravity and even in the dark, i.e., in the absence of visual information. As the animal moved about and especially when it changed direction, the otoliths of the vestibular apparatus moved as a result of the acceleration produced and indirectly stimulated the cells of the hippocampus. The vestibular apparatus therefore intervenes, but gravity plays no role in this particular case.

- Another very simple but very enlightening experiment was performed during the Neurolab mission and showed that the brain was capable of adapting very quickly to weightlessness while conserving its normal reaction capacities for some time. This was demonstrated by a simple gesture such as catching a ball. On the first few trials with a ball released from a spring-loaded device, the astronaut reacted as he would on the ground, that is to say, he reacted thinking that the movement of the ball was going to be pulled downward by the force of gravity. He, therefore, raised his arm too soon. However, after a few trials, the memorization of the effects of gravity disappeared, and the astronaut raised his arm at the right time to catch the ball.

- The notion of internal representation of gravity is particularly interesting. This was shown in an experiment conducted by B. Cohen and G. Clement. On the ground, a man sitting in the dark on a centrifuge giving a transversal or lateral acceleration of 1 g, i.e., equal to gravity, has the sensation of being tilted at an angle of 45°. This orientation corresponds to the resulting force between gravity, which is oriented downward, and the centrifugal force, which is horizontal. Placed under the same conditions on the Columbia shuttle, the astronaut was only subjected to the centrifugal force. After a few days, the astronaut had the feeling of being in the horizontal position as if he were lying on his side on a bed. Under such conditions,

the axis of his head, which goes through both his ears, has the same
direction as the force of gravity. The human brain, therefore, has an
internal representation of gravity that causes him, in the absence of gravity
or any visual information, to interpret a 1 g force as being that of gravity.

A SHORT COURSE IN COMPARATIVE
ANATOMY AND PHYSIOLOGY

Equilibrium is not a unique feature of man or even vertebrates. It already operates
at the cellular level and can be observed in organisms as simple as invertebrates.

The universality of the balance function has led scientists to study the behavior
of various species under conditions of weightlessness. Adult fish onboard Skylab
did not swim normally but rather made frequent loop-like rotational movements.
After a few days, their swimming pattern returned to normal. On the other hand,
alevins that had been born under weightlessness immediately began to swim normally. A Japanese researcher confirmed this phenomenon with the Medaka soft-
water fish: the alevins, born under weightlessness during the IML2 mission of the
American shuttle swam perfectly normally. It is true, however, that the adults of the
same species studied under parabolic flying conditions had never exhibited the
curious looping swimming pattern observed with other species. This merely illustrates that generalization is difficult in biology!

Another experiment conducted on amphibians during a seven-day space flight
clearly showed the adaptation capacity of the vestibular apparatus. Gualtierotti, an
Italian-American scientist, placed two toads in an aquarium equipped with a rotational device that provided a gravitational force of about 0.5 g. He measured the
vestibular activity by recording the nervous influx along the vestibular nerve. This
experiment showed that after two or three days of disturbed activity, normal
responses to acceleration or rest returned.

Finally, it is worth ending this chapter by mentioning an original experiment
that was thought of by a 17-year-old student from Lexington High School in Mas-
sachusetts. Judith Miles started with the idea that spiders must use gravity in order
to spin their webs. When they suspend themselves from a thread, they generate a
plumb line because of their weight. They can then spin a web in a regular pattern.
Judith Miles proposed that NASA study the behavior of the spider under weightlessness. Her project was accepted and the experiment was performed onboard
Skylab by the astronaut Garriott (Figure 30).

Two common spiders, answering to the pretty names of Arabella and Anita, were
used. These animals can live for three weeks without food as long as they have
access to water. They were placed in flasks containing wet sponges. Garriott had to
make them go one after the other into a lit glass chamber while a camera registered
their behavior.

What did the two spiders do? At first, they refused to go into the observation
chamber: Garriott had to force them in! Then, after having suspended themselves
in a corner, they started spinning a web. However, in the absence of gravity, the
results were rather mediocre and yielded an irregular sketch of a web. Two or three

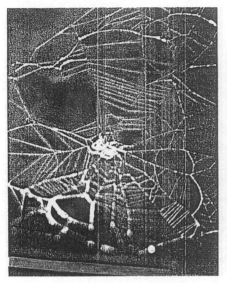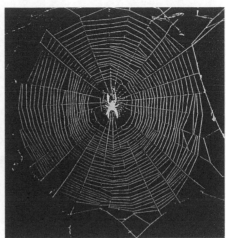

FIGURE 30 *Spider webs and gravity*

Judith Miles, a young American student, thought that spiders might use gravity as an orientation vector when spinning a web. Indeed, during the first days of weightlessness aboard Skylab, the spider spun an irregular web (left) but, after a few days, it adapted to weightlessness and spun a normal web (right).

days later, however, everything was different: Arabella and Anita spun beautiful webs comparable to the ones they made on Earth. They, too, had adapted to weightlessness. Moreover, they adapted so well that they also smartly secreted thinner and, therefore, less resistant thread than they would have done on Earth. Unfortunately, after having devoured two tiny pieces of filet mignon, they refused to drink the water being offered to them and died before the end of the flight. But the experiment the young student had thought of had been successful!

9 The Other Effects of Weightlessness

The cardiovascular, vestibular and musculoskeletal systems are disturbed during a space flight. Because gravity plays a determining role in their functional activity on Earth, the changes observed in weightlessness are therefore not surprising. However, the influence of weightlessness does not limit itself to the above three systems. Indeed, the redistribution of the blood mass created by weightlessness and the resulting changes in blood circulation could have repercussions on organs the activity of which is considered gravity independent. Other reactions occurring during space flights might therefore be linked not to a direct but to indirect effects of weightlessness. However, caution should be exercised before making such connections because the mechanisms causing the appearance of these responses remain unknown.

BLOOD AND WEIGHTLESSNESS

The human body contains 5 liters of blood that is made up of a liquid known as plasma (serum and proteins such as fibrinogen) and a cellular component made of red blood cells, or erythrocytes, and white blood cells or leukocytes. The major content of erythrocytes is a red pigment called haemoglobin each molecule of which contains four iron atoms. Red blood cells transport oxygen to the various organs by binding one oxygen atom to each iron atom. Leukocytes comprise polynuclear cells, lymphocytes and monocytes, as well as platelets, or thrombocytes, which play an important role in blood clotting. Blood platelets are cellular fragments rather than actual cells. A cubic millimeter of blood contains on average 4.5 to 5 million erythrocytes, 6,000 to 8,000 leukocytes and 300,000 thrombocytes.

Blood cells have a limited life span, which is sometimes very short; polynuclear cells and platelets, for instance, merely live a few days. The life span of lymphocytes is variable, lasting from a few days to several years. Red blood cells disappear after 120 days. The destruction of blood cells takes place either in the blood or in the connective tissue of certain organs, which is the case for white blood cells. Platelets and red blood cells are destroyed in the liver and spleen. The destruction of aged erythrocytes causes the degradation of their haemoglobin. The released iron is reused while the rest is degraded into a pigment known as bilirubin in the intestines. The death of old blood cells is compensated by the production of new ones. This cellular renewal is enormous, involving the death and production of 8 to 10 billion red blood cells per hour. As for other blood cells, 300 million polynuclear cells and 100 billion blood platelets are removed and produced per hour. Blood cells are produced in haematopoietic organs: the thymus for certain lymphocytes and the bone marrow for red blood cells, polynuclear cells, platelets and other lymphocytes. All come from large undifferentiated cells, or stem cells of which each organism contains a determined stock. When stem cells divide, two kinds of progeny are produced: an identical cell and a second cell that becomes a committed progenitor, i.e., a cell that will evolve along a particular pathway. In the bone marrow, for example, some cells give rise to red blood cells (after numerous divisions) while others are destined to become polynuclear cells or platelets. When they mature, blood cells leave the organ where they were formed and migrate into the bloodstream. Red blood cells are an exception in that they are still immature when they leave the bone marrow; immature red cells, called reticulocytes, make up about 1% of all red blood cells. Reticulocytes mature rapidly and are transformed into adult red blood cells in about 24 hours. Stem cells can be collected from bone marrow samples, usually by puncturing the sternum. When cultivated in the laboratory, they continue to proliferate and give rise to small colonies from which differentiate blood cells are formed.

Blood cell formation, or hematopoiesis, is influenced by numerous regulating factors. For example, vitamin B12 found in meat, eggs and dairy products stimulates the production of red blood cells. Ionizing radiation, such as X and gamma rays produced by cobalt bombs, have a harmful effect, especially on cells produced in the bone marrow. Erythropoietin, a hormone produced by the kidney and discussed later in this section, stimulates erythropoiesis. Its secretion depends on the oxygen content in the blood. At high altitudes where there is little oxygen, blood is also oxygen-depleted, a phenomenon that is compensated by the production of an abnormally high number of red blood cells thanks to a higher secretion of erythropoietin.

THE EFFECTS OF SPACE FLIGHTS

"Space anemia," reported on Gemini, Apollo, Skylab and Shuttle flights, as well as in cosmonauts aboard the Salyut and Mir space stations, is a reduction in the total red blood cell mass. In standard medicine, anemia is detected by counting red blood cells, measuring the hemoglobin concentration in the blood and by hematocrit measurement. This technique consists of centrifuging a volume of blood in a small graduated test tube to cause the red blood cells and other cells to separate from plasma. The heavier red blood cells sediment at the bottom, and the fraction they constitute is called the hematocrit. Its value varies between 40 and 50%, with an average of 47% in men and 42% in women. It is lower in cases of anemia. For astronauts, however, these methods are not suitable and could lead to erroneous results since weightlessness causes a redistribution of the blood mass as well as plasma loss during the first hours of flight, thereby reducing total blood volume. Under such conditions, a simple count might give the impression that the number of red blood cells is abnormally high. Similarly, studying the blood only by hematocrit measurement could lead to misinterpretations since the hematocrit of astronauts is usually normal, even when increases or reductions of up to 14% in total globular mass have been observed after long missions in space.

To determine the true effects of weightlessness, it is best to calculate the total number of red blood cells in the organism rather than their number per cubic millimeter of blood. In practice, the RBC count is calculated more precisely from the hematocrit and plasma volume measurements. For simplicity, the globular mass is expressed as a volume and is usually around 30 milliliters per kilogram of body weight.

Space anemia thus corresponds to a reduction in total RBC mass. The latter was reduced by 9% after 10 days aboard Spacelab-1 and by 15% after a mission of several weeks. The anemia persists after the flight, with the RBC count recovering its normal value only after about 6 weeks, and sometimes even 3 months, as was the case for Skylab astronauts. Can weightlessness explain the appearance of space anemia? Indeed, a ground simulation experiment lasting 10 days—the same as a shuttle flight—led to a reduction in the RBC count though less pronounced since it was only 4.6%. Simulation experiments with animals using the suspended rat technique produced similar results.

If weightlessness thus appears to be responsible for space anemia, the question is by what mechanism: anemia may be the result of an increase in erythrocyte destruction or a decrease in their production. However, the hypothesis of a combined action cannot be rejected, and many studies have been performed on animals and human beings to test this. In rats, a study carried out on labeled erythrocytes (after uptake of ^{14}C-labeled glycine, a radioactive amino acid), showed that red blood cell destruction was three times greater in animals having flown aboard Cosmos-782 than in the control group of rats. This result is certainly linked to weightlessness as the responses partially disappeared in rats placed in a 1-g centrifuge during the flights (a centrifuge that simulates terrestrial gravity). On the other hand, a reduced red blood cell production seems unlikely since the number of stem cells in the bone marrow was not significantly modified. The number of stem cells was determined by the number of cellular colonies that developed *in vitro* from samples of bone marrow taken from rats flown aboard the Soviet Biosatellite—2044 for 14 days. Levels of erythropoietin, the hormone that regulates erythropoiesis, also remained unchanged.

In humans, erythropoiesis experiments carried out by C. P. A. Alfrey on the shuttle flights provide evidence that anemia in astronauts is due mainly to a lower production of red blood cells. Indeed:

- The production of red blood cells was first studied by measuring the amount of iron used by bone marrow cells. When radioactive iron (^{59}Fe) is injected and blood samples are taken over a period of time the rate of disappearance of this element from plasma can be calculated. This rate is obviously going to increase when erythropoiesis is more active. Now, the remaining volume of unused ^{59}Fe in the astronauts' plasma, measured two hours after the injection, was much higher than in preflight controls.
- Another method consists of taking blood samples from each astronaut and labeling red blood cells *in vitro* with radioactive chromium (^{51}Cr), which has the property of binding to hemoglobin. Once reinjected into the body, the labeled red blood cells will mix with the others. A new sample expresses the proportion of labeled red blood cells. The samples collected later show that their percentage decreases over time. This more or less rapid phenomenon depends on the survival capacity of red blood cells and on the quantity of new cells produced after injection. Here are a few explanations on this point:

- The time it takes for all radioactive red blood cells to disappear shows the life span of these cells (usually 120 days).
- The repeated measurements of chromium level calculated per gram of hemoglobin in the blood yields the production rate of red blood cells. Indeed, a greater level of erythropoiesis leads to an increased quantity of newly synthesized hemoglobin and a consequently more rapid decrease in the level of ^{51}Cr per gram of hemoglobin.

It is important to go into such detail because the results obtained from this method are clear. They show that space anemia in man is not due to an increased destruction of red blood cells, which would lead to a decrease in RBC life span, but rather to a slower production of RBC.

This anemia-producing mechanism can also be confirmed by measuring the level of erythropoietin. This type of measurement, which is more precise nowadays because of extremely sensitive radioimmunoassay techniques, has shown that the level of erythropoietin decreases after the 24th hour of flight, and can be down by 30 to 40% on the third day compared to preflight levels. Such a low secretion rate has repercussions on progenitor cells committed to become red blood cells, i.e., on stem cells already engaged in this cell lineage. Lacking in hormonal stimulus, these cells can no longer divide and die, provoking a reduction in erythropoiesis.

Even if the entire mechanism behind the appearance of space anemia is not yet understood, the effects of weightlessness on erythropoiesis are also demonstrated by the following observations:

- The appearance of abnormally shaped red blood cells, which are known as echinocytes because they have spikes and more or less resemble sea urchins, is proof of a disturbance in erythropoiesis.
- There is a decrease in the level of reticulocytes. As we have seen, this name is given to red blood cells that have not reached maturation yet have already been released from the bone marrow into the bloodstream. These elements contain a narrow filamentous network detected after adding a methylene blue dye and their normal level is very low (below 1% of all red blood cells). This level increases when erythropoiesis increases, as observed for example, after heavy bleeding. The proportion of reticulocytes in astronauts always diminishes, by up to 60%, as was observed during the Spacelab-1 flight. This phenomenon is obviously in line with the smaller production of red blood cells mentioned earlier.

The modifications observed in the red blood cell population are the most remarkable of the disturbances created in blood cells during space flights. Other effects have been reported, however, on polymorphonuclear leucocytes also known as granulocytes because of the presence of granules with various staining properties. Among these cells (neutrophils, eosinophils and basophils), neutrophils are slightly elevated in number while the percentage of eosinophils decreases. The percentage of another class of leucocytes, the lymphocytes, and especially T lymphocytes, also decreases. Contrary to lymphocytes, the percentage of monocytes, which constitute the largest white blood cell subpopulation, is slightly increased. All these modifications, observed principally on returning to Earth, disappear very quickly.

In this case stress probably plays an important role. It has indeed been known for some time that stress affects blood cells, especially lymphocytes and monocytes. There may be other intervening factors during space flights. Nevertheless, the modifications observed in the leucocyte population raise an additional question: as all these cells participate in the defense mechanism of the body against foreign elements, what becomes of the immune response in weightlessness?

THE IMMUNE RESPONSE AND WEIGHTLESSNESS

All vertebrates have an immune system that participates in the defense of the organism against attacks from infectious elements such as viruses, bacteria, fungi and foreign molecules, especially large-sized macromolecules. Confronted with such attacks, the organism can react in two different ways that will be described briefly:

- First, it can destroy foreign elements such as bacteria thanks to polynuclear leucocytes. These cells migrate through capillary walls. Their membrane invaginates around the bacteria and pinches off to form a vesicle inside the cell. Later the enzymes in the vesicle degrade the bacteria. This process is known as phagocytosis. Polynuclear cells can also destroy bacteria by attacking their walls with an enzyme called lysozyme. Other cells, such as macrophages, are also capable of phagocytosis. Macrophages are slightly differentiated cells present in numerous organs such as the liver and lymph nodes. Blood monocytes can also act like macrophages.
- Second, an organism can react using its highly complex immune system where lymphocytes play an essential role. Lymphocytes react each time they encounter a foreign element carrying on its surface particular molecules known as antigens. This is notably the case for bacteria and viruses. With macromolecules, it is usual for only part of the molecule to act as an antigen.

There are two broad classes of immune responses elicited by two different cell populations: B lymphocytes ("B" cells) produced in the bone marrow, and T lymphocytes ("T" cells) produced in the thymus. The thymus is a gland situated in the lower part of the neck and the upper part of the mediastinum, the area between the two lungs. B and T lymphocytes migrate to the blood stream and are found in different parts of the body, among which are the lymph nodes.

Although the immune response uses two different pathways, the starting point is always the same. When infectious agents penetrate the organism, they will attach themselves to the surface of macrophages or monocytes via their antigens. These cells then start to synthesize a particular protein, interleukine, which penetrates the lymphocytes that have gathered at the surface of monocytes or macrophages. In the first type of immunity, known as humoral immunity, B lymphocytes are activated by this process. They become enlarged, lose their differentiation and behave like young cells, once again capable of division. Finally, these lymphocytes transform themselves and become plasma cells, which synthesize antibodies. The latter are proteins called immunoglobulins. There are many varieties, each one specific for a given antigen. The antibodies then migrate into the bloodstream, bond with the corresponding antigens and kill the bacteria carrying the antigen.

The second type of immune response is the cell-mediated immune response. In this case, interleukine activates T lymphocytes, thus provoking their division. These cells then give rise to several varieties of lymphocytes, for instance, natural killer or NK cells, so called because they attach themselves to target cells and kill them.

Many cell types are involved in these highly complex reactions: a class of T cells, called "helpers," produces interleukine-2, which activates other T cells and monocytes. Other lymphocytes, as well as other cells throughout the organism, produce interferon, which is a type of protein molecule capable of attacking viruses. Macrophages also participate in the production of complement, an enzymatic complex capable of activating the immune system and stimulating the phagocytosis of bacteria by polynuclear cells. The activation of lymphocytes, an essential step in the immune response, can be reproduced in the laboratory by placing lymphocytes in the presence of different activating substances such as phytohemagglutinin. The reactivation of lymphocytes can be tested by the resulting lymphoblastic transformation which measures the reaction capacity of the immune system.

THE EFFECTS OF SPACE FLIGHTS

This brief overview provides a basic understanding of the studies made on human beings during space flights. These studies are important since the modifications of the immune response could lead to an increase in infectious events and thereby compromise the success of a mission. For example, on November 21, 1985, the Soviet cosmonaut Vladimir Vasyoutine had to be rushed back to Earth because of a serious infection after more than five months aboard Salyut-7. The infection disappeared rapidly after his return to Earth.

The immune function has been studied during many space missions, and in many cases the results have been variable and nonsignificant, notably the measurements of the level of lysozyme (an enzyme which destroys the bacterial cell wall), complement and various immunoglobulins. During shuttle flights lasting approximately one week, a slight increase in the level of IgG and IgD immunoglobulins was observed but did not exceed normal limits. In other cases, however, some very interesting results were obtained. Indeed, Hungarian and Soviet scientists observed a hypersecretion of interferon in mouse lymphocytes cultivated aboard Soyuz and Salyut. The interferon level was ten times higher than that produced in ground-based experiments. On the other hand, the lymphocytes isolated from cosmonauts immediately after recovery produced four times less interferon than before the flight. The secretion level was once again normal when their lymphocytes were tested six days later. Thus there seems to be a clear difference between *in vitro* and *in vivo* studies. The reduction in interferon secretion observed in astronauts suggests that immune responsiveness is altered under microgravity. Other studies seem to lead to the same conclusion.

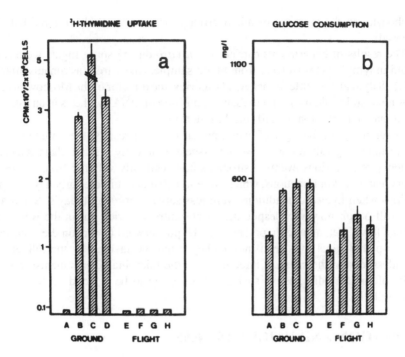

FIGURE 31 *Evidence of the effect of weightlessness at the cellular level*

Exposure of human lymphocytes to weightlessness results in a dramatic decrease in radioactive thymidine intake (a base used in DNA synthesis) and in lower glucose consumption. (Cogoli A. *et al.* experiment, Ecole Polytechnique, Zurich.)

Indeed the activation of lymphocytes was tested *in vitro* after Apollo and Skylab flights, as well as onboard the Salyut and Mir space stations and the Space Shuttle. In many cases, the results pointed to a decrease in the immune response. A reduction of about 75% was observed on the Shuttle flights, but of only 3% in the astronauts on the Spacelab D-1 missions. It was this finding that pushed the Swiss scientist Augusto Gogoli to conduct the same test during the Shuttle flight but on lymphocytes collected before launch (Figure 31). Phytohemagglutinin was added in order to induce cell activation, as well as radioactive thymidine (used in DNA synthesis). The results were spectacular: the lymphocytes were practically incapable of incorporating thymidine, suggesting that weightlessness could inhibit lymphocyte activation and, consequently, DNA synthesis and proliferation. Later, ground experiments demonstrated that hypergravity had the opposite effect. Cogoli and his colleagues have subsequently shown that the inhibition of lymphocytes in weightlessness disappears if the cells are cultivated in an environment containing plastic microcarrier beads. The lymphocytes and monocytes attach themselves to this substrate and can then make contact with one another. The interleukin produced by the monocytes can cross the lymphocyte membrane and induce cellular activation. This suggests that microgravity acts only by indirect rather than direct effect. However, caution is recommended when interpreting these results since more recent experiments have shown that the activation of lymphocytes in the presence of microcarrier beads was not only restored but even increased.

The results of experiments carried out *in vitro* during space flights were found to hold in lymphocytes isolated from blood samples taken from astronauts after the Skylab, Salyut and Shuttle flights. A.I. Grigoriev, the director of the Moscow Institute of Biomedical Problems, found the same inhibition of DNA synthesis in an astronaut after a one-year mission aboard the Mir station.

In summary, in the light of experimental research results, the immune system appears to undergo alterations in weightlessness. Clinically, it seems there is a higher frequency of infectious events. Astronauts have certainly suffered from cutaneous, urinary, ear and skin infections, which were more frequent in the early days of space missions when hygienic conditions were less satisfactory than today's. Small accidents still occur, however, despite the strict controls carried out in the weeks preceding a flight. Yet, another hypothesis can be put forward to explain the occurrence of such pathological incidents: indeed they might be favored by the influence of weightlessness on the cause of infection, i.e., the microbial agents themselves. The results of some studies, as we shall see later, seem to be in good agreement with this possibility.

RESPIRATION AND WEIGHTLESSNESS

Lungs deliver oxygen from the air and draw out the carbon dioxide (CO_2), the waste resulting from cell metabolism in the human body. These exchanges take place in the 300 million alveoli, which are small sacs filled with air, the membranes of which house an important capillary network. Exchanges between blood and air take place in the alveolar wall. Blood from the pulmonary arteries flows into the capillary network then continues into venules leading to pulmonary veins. Unlike other blood vessels, the pulmonary artery transports CO_2-rich blood whereas pulmonary veins contain oxygen-rich blood. Oxygen and CO_2 are attached to hemoglobin in red blood cells.

With each breath a human being takes, approximately 500 cm^3 of air moves in and out of the lungs. This is known as the tidal volume. A deeper breath can increase inspiration and expiration; the amount of air that can be inhaled and exhaled is then increased by nearly 1.1 liters, respectively. The amount of air known as the inspiration reserve volume is 2.9 liters. Conversely, the 1.1 liters exhaled beyond a normal breath are known as the expiratory reserve volume. The residual volume is the amount of air that cannot be expelled, regardless of the effort. The deepest breath possible—the combination of the tidal volume, the inspiration reserve and the expiration reserve volumes—is referred to as the vital capacity (~4 to 5 liters). Respiration occurs thanks to the movement of the diaphragm (the wall that separates the abdomen from the thorax) as well as the ribcage movements induced by intercostal muscle contraction.

Gravity on Earth affects respiration. In the vertical position, the intestines do not exert pressure on the diaphragm and the pulmonary volume—the residual air volume especially—increases. The opposite occurs in the horizontal position. Posture also modifies the ribcage movement, thereby causing changes in the depth of breathing.

On the other hand, gravity is responsible for the structural and functional heterogeneity of the lungs as well, thereby creating a true gradient. Blood perfusion and respiratory exchanges are thus greater in the lower region than in the upper, or apical, part of the lungs. In this region, the alveoli are at rest, more expanded, relatively less inflated than those in the lower-lung area and therefore participate less in respiration. These data demonstrate the relevance of studying respiratory physiology under microgravity.

Before Gagarin's flight, there were serious fears concerning the influence of microgravity as it was suspected that the redistribution of blood in the ribcage area might give rise to a pulmonary edema with serious consequences on the astronaut's survival. As it turns out, astronauts apparently breathe normally in space, which does not mean, however, that the absence of gravity has no effect on respiration. Indeed studies carried out during the Spacelab and Shuttle flights have revealed a decrease of approximately 10% in the tidal volume and the vital capacity during the first stages of a flight. After one to eight days, on the other hand, one can observe an increase in lung functional capacity, i.e., the amount of gas that passes through the alveolar membrane per minute. Furthermore, space investigations suggest that pulmonary heterogeneity does not entirely disappear.

OTHER MANIFESTATIONS

Excluding the different systems the functional activity of which depends more or less directly on gravity, and apart from blood and the immune system, weightlessness does not appear to cause important changes in the rest of the body. Nor does it have a noticeable effect on the digestive system, although intestinal transit time often seems slightly slower.

Also of interest is the astronauts' sleep–wake cycle, one of the most spectacular manifestations of circadian rhythms. Circadian rhythms last approximately 24 hours and affect a large number of an organism's functions. These functions are linked for the most part to genuine internal clocks, which are located in the nerve centers and are continuously set right by the change from day to night. It is difficult to account for the periodic functioning of these clocks, which may be controlled by several factors. As space flights take men greater distances away from Earth, one might expect some of these factors and consequently certain biological rhythms to be affected. This possibility has led to research on lower organisms. One experiment performed aboard the shuttle Columbia on *Neurospora*, a mushroom that develops spores according to a 24-hour rhythm, showed that the flight had caused only a slight lengthening in the spore production cycle, indicating the circadian rhythm had been virtually preserved. The same conclusion was drawn from an experiment involving *Actinomyces*, another mushroom with a growth subject to periodic variations.

In astronauts, space flights seem to have no effect on circadian rhythms either, or at least on sleeping patterns during short-term missions. In the majority of cases, Russian cosmonauts sleep normally, although some do occasionally resort to sleeping medication since their sleep is disturbed by very active schedules (and by the yearning to contemplate the Earth from an altitude of more than 200 km!). However, close analysis has revealed the existence of minor disruptions during a particular phase of each sleep cycle—there are several cycles per night—known as paradoxical sleep. This phase of the sleep cycle manifests itself by continued brain activity, as electroencephalograms and rapid eye movements show. Recordings made on Spacelab astronauts suggest that the relative duration of paradoxical sleep is doubled, with this phase of sleep corresponding more or less to a quarter of the duration of sleep. The frequency of eye movement also appears to increase. All these phenomena decrease after a few days, which again points to the capacity of the human organism to adapt to the space environment. Nevertheless, it is impossible to conclude that stays of increasing length in space will not gradually alter circadian rhythms and in particular the sleep–wake cycles, which could be of concern for future long-term manned missions.

Astronauts' sensory activity is also noteworthy, because whereas hearing, smell and taste appear to function normally, vision seems to be modified in that visual acuity from great distances is improved. On one of the early flights, Gordon Cooper reported he could see the movement of cars from an altitude of 80 kilometers. Edward White, the second American to undertake an EVA, said he could make out roads, ship wakes and lines of street lamps from his Gemini space capsule. In general, linear-shaped objects are the clearest, and this apparent improvement in eyesight might only be due to the particular observation conditions from above the Earth's atmosphere. Indeed measurements taken by both the Americans and the Soviets have not revealed any improvement in visual acuity. As a matter of fact, the opposite has been shown, since astronauts appear to suffer from decreased visual acuity and perceive distant objects inside the ship's cabin with more difficulty. This functional short-sightedness, also observed in submarine crews, could be linked to confinement and monotonous surroundings. It is also interesting to note that astronauts confined to the dark report experiencing strange luminous sensations or white flashes, the origin of which will be addressed in the chapter dealing with the effects of cosmic radiation on living organisms.

CONCLUSION

Although astronauts appear to live normally and accomplish their duties efficiently on a mission, the truth is that weightlessness does provoke disturbances in the human body. In addition to modifications in blood distribution and a reduction in blood mass, astronauts are subject to disturbances in equilibrium, bone demineralization, muscular atrophy and anemia … a long and varied list.

In spite of this, it is possible to survive and even live fairly normally thanks to regulating or compensating mechanisms. In the cardiovascular apparatus for example, the apparent overloading of blood in the body gives rise to a whole series of neuroendocrine responses. Space research and ground simulation experiments have indeed increased our knowledge on this subject by showing that the volemia regulating mechanism described by J. P. Henry-Gauer is not valid in humans. Regarding body equilibrium, sight replaces proprioception and the otolithic system to a large extent, since these are at rest for the most part. There again, experiments in space have provided important results by proving that nerve centers can adapt. This neuronal plasticity is a major concept in nerve physiology. In addition, bone demineralization, muscular atrophy and even space anemia are perhaps not as serious as they might appear at first since weightlessness places the astronaut in a new environment in which mechanical constraints are absent. Standing upright, moving around and displacing objects are much less of an effort for an astronaut in space. The need to have such a resistant skeleton, developed musculature and rich blood supply disappears, and muscles no longer require as much nutrition and oxygen as they do on Earth.

This capacity to adapt is also illustrated by the fact that an organism's responses to weightlessness evolve during the different phases of flight, just as they do during simulation experiments. For instance, the space sickness that appears during the first hours of weightlessness usually disappears within two to three days. Losses of plasma and electrolytes, for instance, potassium, are an immediate result of blood mass redistribution but decrease after a few days of flight. Space anemia, which appears during the first weeks, stabilizes after 30 to 45 days.

To sum up the situation, accepting a certain number of hypotheses and extrapolating somewhat, one can draw curves to show physiological variations as a function of time. In doing this, one can see that the curves first rise more or less abruptly and early (Figure 32). Then, after a few days, or sometimes one or two weeks, the curves tend to fall off to form pointed or rounded bell shapes before finally leveling off to a plateau after a few days or as much as one and a half months, depending

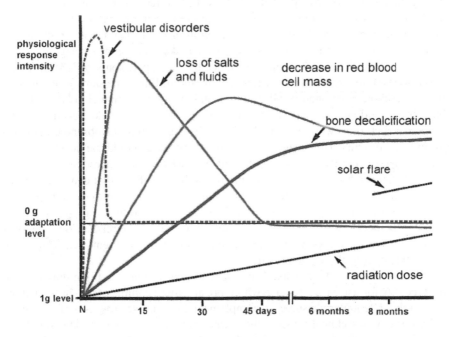

FIGURE 32 *Time course of physiological responses during the different phases of a space flight*

Body systems can adapt to microgravity, but the curves showing the physiological responses reach a plateau situated above the normal level (1 g). In another words, most physiological systems reach a new steady state, which differs from the state of homeostasis (physiological equilibrium) before the flight.

on the case. However, this does not mean a return to the starting point, to a state of equilibrium or homeostasis as usually happens on Earth. In fact, to take but a few significant examples, while plasma loss actually stops, volemia in astronauts remains lower than normal. The nerve centers of the vestibular system acquire new automated programs; muscles have a new structural organization; the total volume of red blood cells remains below normal values. The curves have become horizontal, but what makes this striking is that the plateau is situated above the normal level. The astronaut has thus adapted to a new environment. He is not quite the same as he was prior to the flight.

This certainly does not imply that adaptation is perfect or that all problems have been resolved. For example, while calcium loss decreases with time it still persists throughout the entire flight. It may take missions lasting several years for the processes of osteogenesis and bone resorption to reach a state of equilibrium. This remains to be elucidated. Similarly, it is impossible to know if the state of equilibrium attained by the other systems will subsist when the length of missions is progressively increased. Although the heart seems to tolerate space conditions so far, myocardium structural changes might eventually lead to serious dysfunction thus jeopardizing the survival of astronauts.

As previously mentioned, the 24-hour sleep–wake cycle is the most remarkable among circadian rhythms. Short flights have little effect on the human biological clock, but the effects of longer missions remain to be determined. In the absence of the usual influence of night and day, a disruption in the normal circadian rhythm of the body, or desynchronosis, occurs. The sleep–wake cycle tends to lengthen, often reaching a periodicity of 48 hours, as shown by the experiments of Michel Siffre, who remained underground for an extended period of time. The same might be true in space. Although astronauts artificially maintain a rhythm identical to that on Earth, there is no evidence to suggest that a long stay in space would not disrupt this biological rhythm as well, with the kind of individual variations observed in underground experiments. This is an important point, because should the desynchronization vary in its onset and magnitude between astronauts, repercussions on their physical and psychological capacities might result in conflicts that could jeopardize the mission. From this perspective, the human capacity to adapt to space is perhaps not as extensive as originally believed. When selecting future astronauts, it may therefore be necessary to measure their ability to maintain circadian rhythms over a period of several weeks when placed in an artificial environment, i.e., without the usual signals from the world outside.

The discovery of the effects of microgravity, the increase in flight duration and the necessity for astronauts to cope with more and more complex tasks have justified the search for "countermeasures" to complement the adaptive processes of the human body. For obvious ethical reasons, these countermeasures will never allow us to know the full effects of weightlessness and the limits of man's capacity to adapt. Furthermore, the role of countermeasures is not only limited to improving man's survival in space. They allow him to readapt to gravity upon his return to Earth and recover a normal equilibrium.

While a large number of problems concerning manned flights have been resolved, this cannot be said about the future. The problems will be different when exploring Mars which will require manned missions lasting about two years. They will be even greater when we imagine a spaceship leaving one day with a few hundred men and women onboard to conquer space in the hope of colonizing perhaps new planets. What will then become of the human organism both from the physiological and psychological point of view? Will it be possible to create artificial gravity? There is no doubt that these men and women, who will never return to Earth, will be different from the *Homo sapiens* that we are. They will have become Spatiopithecus creatures!

Coming back to Earth and considering the near future, physicians, scientists and engineers confronted with the prospect of manned missions of increasing duration and frequency have a dual role. First, they have to ensure the survival of astronauts in weightlessness and their readaption upon returning to Earth. Second, they must improve our basic knowledge in the field of human physiology with further research. This is without doubt an arduous task since research in space physiology and medicine is still in its early stages.

SPIN-OFFS FOR STANDARD MEDICINE

The benefits of space research are not limited to space. Indeed, the space program has led to the development of medical techniques and equipment that are nowadays commonly used on Earth. Although this goes beyond the scope of this book, a few examples will be given to demonstrate the existence of such applications.

Research performed in the United States and the Soviet Union in preparation of manned flights has improved the physiological monitoring of the human body and the methods currently used in surgery and cardiology.

NASA developed a small apparatus that can be implanted in the human body to reduce auricular fibrillation, a particularly serious cardiac rhythm anomaly. One spin-off of miniaturization technology developed for satellites and the Viking missions to Mars has been the manufacture of small, implantable perfusion pumps which, given impulses, automatically deliver medications such as insulin, as required. The Holter monitor, used a great deal in cardiology, was developed in part for Skylab missions, as were sonographs, which have been increasingly miniaturized thanks to space research. The ophthalmological use of lasers in the treatment of detached retina was also perfected at the NASA Ames Research Center. New medical equipment was also developed in other fields such as ophthalmology and otorhinolaryngology.

The few examples above illustrate that space medical research is not only geared to ensuring the survival of human beings in space but also to improving fundamental knowledge in physiology and biology. It is important to remember that this type of research also produces new developments in biotechnology, which is commonly used in medicine and biology nowadays.

10 Space Cell Biology

Gravity and weightlessness affect blood and others tissues, the mass and volume of which are substantial. It is not surprising that it should exert an influence on small organelles with a higher density than that of the medium in which they are suspended: this is, for instance, the case for otoliths in the utricle and saccule and for amyloplasts in plant cells.

What happens, however, in the case of cells no larger than a few dozen micrometers in diameter? For some, the answer is simple: there is no or at least no significant effect. Should we therefore consider the question answered once and for all or should we attempt to investigate the matter further?

To dismiss the usefulness of more research in this area would show a lack of seriousness and might comfort the sceptics in their ignorance of the results reported below. It is important to point out that the study of the effects of gravity and weightlessness at the cellular level is of great interest to both biologists and physicians. Indeed, reactions observed in man, such as changes in the immune response, might result from the addition of a number of modifications at the cellular level. Similarly, it is quite possible that part of the bone modifications observed on orbital flights could result from a direct action of microgravity on the cells responsible for bone tissue formation and resorption.

Current knowledge about the effects of gravity on cells is based on both theoretical arguments and actual results from space research.

THE THEORETICAL ARGUMENTS

Theoretically, the influence of gravity is negligible at the molecular level and notably in the cytoplasm because the forces that bind molecules together are infinitely greater than those exerted by gravity. The problem is different for organelles that have a slightly greater density than that of the cytoplasm. Thus gravity-induced effects could appear for the nucleus (Figure 33), which is relatively large (about 10 micrometers in diameter), and might also be expected to do so for organelles such as mitochondria. However, nothing precipitates inside the cell. The latter has a three-dimensional architecture even though its structure might be expected to be unstable due to constant molecular movements and cytoplasmic streaming. While cell structure is probably maintained through the action of various factors, the main actor is no doubt the cytoskeleton. The latter is a network of very thin filaments (microfilaments) and narrow tubes (microtubules) made up of proteins called actin and tubulin, respectively. These extend throughout the cell but are more concentrated around the nucleus and just beneath the cell membrane. The actin and tubulin protein molecules are composed of subunits that rapidly join and separate inside the cell. Among its multiple functions, the cytoskeleton maintains the shape of the cell, and its presence should therefore

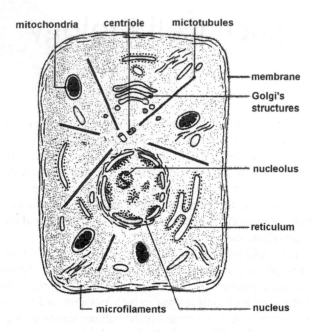

FIGURE 33 *Diagram of a mammalian cell*

The cell is surrounded by a membrane and contains a usually approximately spherical nucleus. The part of the cell around the nucleus is called the cytoplasm. Inside the cytoplasm, the cell contains many organelles such as mitochondria, endoplasmic reticulum vesicles, microfilaments and microtubules.

counterbalance the influence of gravity. Gravity can also affect cells through convection phenomena. Indeed, convection phenomena appear all the time since metabolism creates zones of higher or lower molecular concentrations and hence density gradients within the cytoplasm. This results in cytoplasmic streaming, which can easily be detected under the microscope in plant cells where it is quite pronounced. In space, these phenomena should stop or at any rate be attenuated because convection, like sedimentation, disappears in weightlessness.

How can gravity and microgravity affect cells? The answer is not easy. Basing himself on the work of Nobel Prize laureate I. Prigogine, D. A. M. Mesland of the ESA has proposed that microgravity acts when the cells, the metabolism of which is never in complete equilibrium, go through states of great instability. The chemical reactions of cellular metabolism are complex, being regulated by vast numbers of enzymes and feedback mechanisms that slow down or block steps in the synthesis of particular compounds when enough has accumulated. These chemical reactions do not develop linearly and can, at certain times, suddenly be pushed in one direction or another. According to Mesland, it is when this happens that cells are highly sensitive to environmental factors and are therefore affected by microgravity. Deprived of the natural gravity factor, cell metabolism and other reactions could develop in unusual directions, thus accounting for the responses observed in space experiments.

It must be pointed out that the results of space experiments could in theory be induced by an indirect effect of microgravity. Indeed, the absence of gravity modifies the distribution of substances in the culture medium since sedimentation disappears in weightlessness. However, present space experimental conditions and the results of experiments performed on Earth, using a slow clinostat to prevent sedimentation, have shown that this hypothesis can be, in most cases, eliminated.

THE RESULTS OF SPACE EXPERIMENTS

CELL DIVISION

Bacteria were investigated on many occasions since the beginning of astronautics. For Mattoni, the proliferation of *Escherichia coli* (*E. coli*) flown aboard the U.S. Biosatellite-2 in 1971 was stimulated. Other researchers observed similar effects with *Proteus vulgaris* and *Bacillus subtilis*. Culturing *E. coli* on seven shuttle flights, D. Kluns reported that the cell proliferation rate had approximately doubled. However, in other experiments, microgravity did not affect the proliferation rate of *E. coli*. This was the case for the results reported by G. Gasset with the *E. coli* cultured on the STS-42 mission. As for Kacena *et al.*, who reported a stimulation effect in several species of bacteria cultured aboard the Mir station, the responses were only due to an indirect effect on the culture medium.

Tixador in Toulouse, France, reported other interesting results from experiments carried out aboard both the Solyut and Shuttle flights. In space, the bacteria are more resistant to antibiotics, a phenomenon probably linked to lower binding of antibiotic molecules to the bacterial membrane (Figure 34).

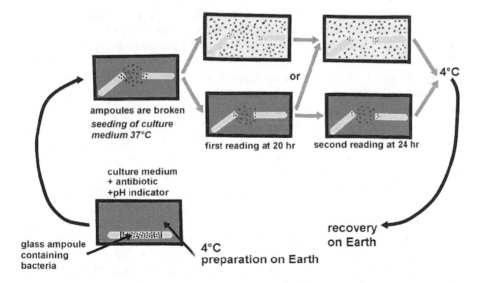

FIGURE 34 *Diagrams illustrating the different steps of the Cytos 2 experiment (see Color figure VI at the of the book)*

Bacteria were placed in glass ampoules. A plastic bag was filled with a colored medium containing an antibiotic. In space, the glass ampoules were broken to let the bacteria grow in the culture medium. The color change in the pH indicator demonstrated that bacteria under microgravity could grow in spite of the presence of antibiotics used at various concentrations (Tixador, R. *et al.*).

Animal and human cells have also been investigated in space. Using special techniques, cells can be cultured in microgravity and made to differentiate, at least in some cases. Indeed, in a well-known experiment, P. O. Montgomery used human pulmonary embryonic fibroblasts, which are weakly differentiated connective tissue cells, and cultivated them for 3 to 11 days aboard Skylab. No modification in growth or structure was detected. Another experiment carried out by a laboratory of the Moscow Academy of Sciences on connective and epithelial hamster cells also provided negative results. The same occurred when carrot cells were cultivated aboard Cosmos-782: the cells divided and differentiated normally. More recently, the proliferation of hamster kidney cells cultivated during the IML-1 Spacelab mission remained unchanged, in agreement with Montgomery's results.

However, these results cannot be extended to all cell types. In particular, the Swiss scientist Augusto Cogoli carried out many experiments on human lymphocytes. In this case, microgravity has a strong inhibiting effect on cell division as shown by the lower uptake of radioactive thymidine, a compound used in DNA synthesis and added to the culture medium during the space flight.

Single-cell organisms such as protozoa have also been investigated in space, particularly in the Franco-Soviet Cytos experiments (Planel, H. *et al.*, 1981). These experiments used *Paramecium*, a protozoan found in fresh water and cultivated for different purposes in many laboratories. The Cytos experiment was prepared at the Institute of Biomedical Problems in Moscow (Figure 35). The cultures were initially kept at low temperature to block cell division, especially during launch when vibrations or acceleration might affect the cells. The cultures were taken to Baikonur and placed aboard Soyuz-6; after docking Soyuz to the Salyut space station, they were transferred to an incubator. Once exposed to a temperature of 25°C, the paramecia were able to divide again. Fifteen culture samples were taken every 12 hours and killed by chemical fixation. The same experiment was carried out on Earth following the same protocol. The results of the Cytos experiment, like those of another performed the following year, were conclusive: the paramecia cultivated in space proliferated more quickly than when cultivated on the ground. Other effects were also noted, such as an increase in cellular volume and a decrease in protein and calcium content. The origin of these responses and especially the higher cell proliferation was studied afterward. The experiment was again performed aboard Spacelab using the Biorack module developed by the ESA. The module was equipped with two small 1 *g* centrifuges allowing the cultures to be submitted to "normal" gravity. The results of this experiment were spectacular since the flight once again stimulated the proliferation of cells cultured in weightlessness while this effect almost totally disappeared in the cultures subjected to a 1 *g* acceleration (Figure 36). These results show that microgravity is largely responsible for changes in cell proliferation and demonstrate that gravity can have an influence at the cellular level (Planel, H. *et al.*, 1986; Richoilley, G. *et al.*, 1986).

This conclusion was later confirmed by studying the effects of hypergravity when placing cultures in a ground-based centrifuge. The proliferation rate decreased when cells were exposed to 5 to 10 *g*. These results are in good agreement with experiments on the green algae *Chlamydomonas* which has a fluctuating metabolic activity and a capacity to proliferate that is significantly increased under weightlessness.

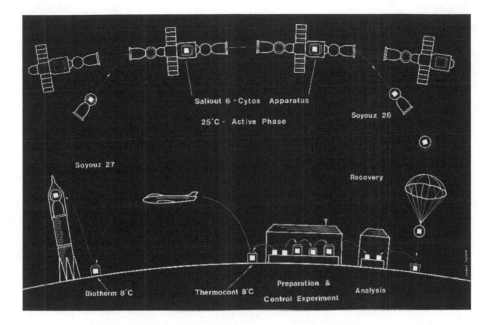

FIGURE 35 *Diagrams illustrating the Cytos experiment*

In a first experiment, cultures of a single-cell organism, *Paramecium,* were placed aboard Soyuz and kept at low temperature. In orbit, cultures were transferred to an incubator kept at 25°C aboard the Soviet station Salyut-6. Cultures were automatically killed by a chemical fixative and investigated after return to Earth aboard a Soyuz spacecraft. A control experiment was performed on Earth according to the same schedule. A similar experiment was carried out later aboard the shuttle during the IML1 mission.

THE CELL MEMBRANE AND EXCHANGES
WITH THE EXTRACELLULAR ENVIRONMENT

The hypothesis that microgravity affects the cell membrane has been raised on several occasions. First of all, continuous exchanges occur across the cell membrane in order to ensure nutrition and respiration. Furthermore, cells are always receiving information from organs like the endocrine glands in the form of ligands, which are chemical compounds that bind to protein receptors located in the membrane. The receptors in turn activate other molecules present in the membrane or in the cytoplasm. This message transmission, which temporarily modifies metabolism or particular cellular functions, is called transduction (this phenomenon will be discussed later). In other cases, ligands and receptors penetrate the cell by a phenomenon called endocytosis. An absence of binding to membrane receptors could explain the effects of microgravity. However, this hypothesis seems unlikely as shown by short-term experiments aboard rocket probes and parabolic flights. Indeed the binding of Concanavalin A or the activator PHA to lymphocyte receptors occurs normally. In the same way, insulin and the cell growth factor EGF bind the membrane receptors of osteosarcoma (malignant bone tumor) cells and penetrate the cytoplasm by endocytosis. These results suggest that the hypothesis whereby gravity exerts an

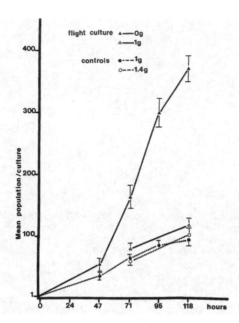

FIGURE 36 *Results of the Paramecium experiment*

The experiment was carried out onboard the shuttle. In-flight cultures show a very significant increase in cell growth, but this effect disappeared when cultures were placed in a 1 *g* centrifuge aboard the shuttle. These curves demonstrate the influence of gravity on the multiplication of a single-cell organism.

influence on the membrane seems unlikely, at least given the current state of knowledge and the experimental conditions used in these studies.

Nevertheless, R. Hemmersbach, among other authors, believes that gravity, which controls the locomotion and spatial orientation of *Paramecium*, affects the potassium and calcium ion channels in the membrane. The swimming of the cell induces hydrostatic pressure differences between the cytoplasm and the medium. This could provoke the opening of ion channels, which in turn regulates the beat of cilia at the surface of the *Paramecium*.

The Cytoskeleton

The cytoskeleton plays an important role in cells. In addition to maintaining cell structure, it also participates in mobility, shape and division. Microtubules reorganize during cell division thus giving rise to the mitotic spindle which guides the migration of chromosomes toward the two future cells. Genes determine the nature of the cytoskeleton, but gravity might affect the distribution of its different elements. Although a precise explanation cannot be given on this subject, some interesting results have already been observed. For instance, tubulin is disorganized and irregularly distributed in muscle cells exposed to simulated microgravity, and a rearrangement of microtubules has been observed in human lymphocytes after a rocket probe flight.

According to James Tabony in Grenoble, France, gravity comes into play during the assembly of the subunits that form microtubules. According to the branching-off concept, microtubules in solution might evolve to give different configurations, a phenomenon in which gravity could play an important role. *In vitro* birefringence studies have shown that microtubular organization varies according to whether the test tube of tubulin solution is tilted at 0°, 45° or 90° with respect to gravity. Can it be concluded that microgravity alters the formation and orientation of microtubules *in vivo*? The fact that cells have to divide normally in the body of astronauts—they would not survive otherwise—shows how difficult it is to apply *in vitro* experimental results to living organisms.

ENERGY METABOLISM

Many experiments carried out on different biological material suggest there is a decrease in energy consumption in weightlessness. On the basis of theoretical considerations, G. W. Nace formulated the hypothesis that this phenomenon occurs under microgravity because cells contain organelles of different density, thereby creating a torque. To maintain their architecture, the cells are normally driven to expend energy, a phenomenon that disappears in space. Montgomery reported a reduction in glucose consumption in the course of an experiment that was long considered negative. The same phenomenon has been found in human lymphocyte cultures and bone models.

A decrease in energy consumption may also explain the results of experiments carried out on *Paramecium*. Under normal environmental conditions, *Paramecium* resists gravity owing to its ability to swim, thereby avoiding sedimentation. The beating of the cilia that cover the cell surface allows the organism to swim but requires energy. *Paramecium* draws energy from the breakdown of ATP (adenosine triphosphate), an energy-rich substance found in all cells, which is also used for cell division. It can be assumed the movements of *Paramecium* are easier in the absence of gravity. The saved ATP might then be used for cell division, thus explaining the higher cell proliferation. To support this theory, ground-based experiments have shown that the ATP level decreases in *Paramecium* exposed to hypergravity and that the opposite occurs in simulated microgravity.

GENES

Genes are composed of DNA molecules that play an essential role in cell metabolism. They are the templates from which messenger RNA (m-RNA) molecules are synthesized. These molecules leave the nucleus to go into the cytoplasm where amino acid molecules bind to the m-RNA. This binding does not occur randomly but depends upon the RNA structure, which is itself a function of the structure of the gene from which it is formed. Later, the amino acids are bound together to form protein molecules. In other words, the genes control RNA synthesis and consequently protein synthesis.

It is difficult to understand the effect of gravity on genes, especially since the number of experiments has been limited so far. Furthermore, although remarkable progress has been achieved in molecular biology, the effects of gravity have never been taken into account in earth-based experiments. Nevertheless, possible effects have been detected in protooncogenes, i.e., genes that regulate cell division and cause cancers to appear when they are transformed into oncogenes. Indeed, the expression of the c-myc protooncogene is increased in human Hela cancer cells exposed to 35 g. The same phenomenon was found in the c-fos protooncogene in human A431 cancer cells. Conversely, simulated microgravity resulted in the opposite phenomenon. Furthermore, R. de Groot in Utrecht, the Netherlands, reported that such gravity-induced effects only occur when cells are in the presence of activating substances like the epithelial growth factor (EGF) or the TPA phorbolester. These compounds bind to membrane receptors and act by signal transduction to stimulate protooncogenes. The pathways of this signal transduction could be affected by gravity, as shown by experiments performed with various activating factors. The influence of gravity has been detected in experiments using EGF or TPA, the transduction pathway of which includes the enzyme protein kinase C (pkC). On the other hand, no gravity-induced effects have been observed with other stimulating factors not involving pkC.

The above investigations suggest that gravity does not act directly on gene expression but on protein kinase C. This conclusion is in agreement with Didier Schmitt and Jason Hatton's studies on the localization of this enzyme. In weightlessness, the pkC level in the nucleus decreases while it increases considerably in the cytoplasm. This interesting result was obtained using leukemia cell lines derived from lymphocytes and monocytes, precisely the cells used in Cogoli's experiments. Gravity also affected pkC in cells, as shown by the decrease in interleukine-1 and -2 monocyte and lymphocyte secretion in weightlessness, this decrease being enhanced when the cells were treated in space with TPA. Now, TPA activates the genes that control interleukine synthesis and, as we have already mentioned, protein kinase C is involved in responses induced by TPA.

Furthermore, enhanced expression of the LDH-A gene was also reported in human renal cells cultured for six days on the shuttle (Hammond *et al.*).

In conclusion, the theoretical arguments in favor of gravity having a direct influence on cells are confirmed by the results of space experiments carried out using different models. Numerous points remain to be elucidated, especially concerning the gravity sensing mechanisms used by cells. The development of astronautics and gravitational biology has opened new fields of research. The results on the influence of different gravitational levels on protooncogenes and pkC certainly present an original and particularly interesting avenue for further studies to be carried out in the ISS.

11 The Effects of Gravity and Weightlessness on Plants

In 1806, a British botanist by the name of Knight conducted the following experiment: he placed a plantule (a germinating seed) on the edge of a horizontal disc made to rotate by a stream of water which also kept the plant humid. When the disc was stationary, the plantule root was directed vertically downwards; when the disk rotated at high speed, the root oriented itself according to the centrifugal force and became horizontal. On the other hand, a lower rotation speed induced the root to take a slanted position as if another force was partially counteracting the centrifugal force. This was the first demonstration that gravity affects the orientation of plant organs. The phenomenon of plant sensitivity to gravity and its consequences were later termed geotropism. This is but one of a number of instances of the influence of external factors on plants. The influence of light or phototropism is another well-known phenomenon.

Geotropism is an essential function found in a very large number of plants. Thanks to it, plants are able to develop according to specific orientations. Its effects, however, differ according to the plant organ under consideration and only roots take their precise orientation according to gravity. This is referred to as positive geotropism. The stems, on the other hand, usually direct themselves vertically upward, and we speak of negative geotropism. Finally, branches and root ramifications grow obliquely.

Supposing the influence of gravity is countered by placing a plantule with its root and stem in a horizontal plane. The plantule recovers its usual orientation within minutes. Thus gravity clearly plays a role as a reference vector, the "plumb line" already mentioned in relation to Man and the animal kingdom.

THE GRAVITROPIC RESPONSE

When a plantule from a lentil seed, for instance, has its root placed in a horizontal position, the root starts curving after 20 minutes, a lapse of time called the latency period. The root continues to curve until it finds itself—after 90 minutes to 2 hours—in the vertical position. The root has, therefore, sensed the influence of gravity. One can say there has been a gravitropic reaction. This phenomenon obviously raises several questions:

What minimum acceleration—in other words what minimum g force value—is required for this reaction to occur? This question can be answered thanks to clinostat experiments.

Supposing a plantule is placed on the horizontal disc of a clinostat, with the root in a vertical position. As the clinostat is made to rotate, a centrifugal force is created which is perpendicular to the vertical rotation axis. The roots now tend to curve to adopt the direction of this centrifugal force. This response appears with an acceleration of about $1.5 \times 10^{-4}\,g$, which demonstrates the remarkable sensitivity of the root to gravity.

- How much time does the gravity-linked stimulation need to operate in order to induce a gravitropic response? As will be seen later, the answer is simple under microgravity. On the ground the answer is obtained by using a slowly rotating clinostat, which makes about one rotation per minute. This counters the effect of gravity, the roots being periodically in the low (normal) or high (inverted) position. As one might have predicted, the root orientation becomes disorderly. Now, if the clinostat is momentarily stopped before resuming its rotation, the roots tend to get oriented vertically, which is evidence for the existence of a gravitropic response. However, the clinostat has to be stopped and thus the plant exposed to gravity for a minimum of about 30 seconds for the response to appear. This value corresponds to the presentation time (minimum time of exposure to gravity required to induce a gravitropic reaction). There again the little plantule exhibits its high sensitivity to the influence of gravity.
- By what mechanism does the gravitropic response occur, and which part of the root is capable of sensing the gravity signal? The answer to this question has been known for a long time: the sensing zone is the root cap, that is to say the extremity of the root, since its removal abolishes the gravitropic response. The root cap contains large cells called statocytes (Figure 37). When growing vertically these cells are polarized, the nucleus

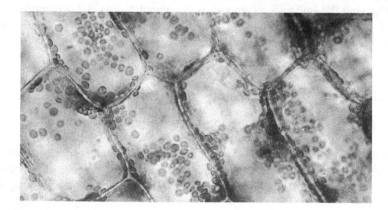

FIGURE 37 *Plant cells (see Color figure VII at the end of the book)*
In many plants, the terminal part of the root contains large cells called statocytes, limited by a thick wall. In addition to the cytoskeleton and endoplasmic reticulum, their cytoplasm contains organelles made up of starch, the amyloplasts or statoliths. Amyloplasts move inside the cell under the influence of gravity. (Pr. G. Perbal, University of Paris.)

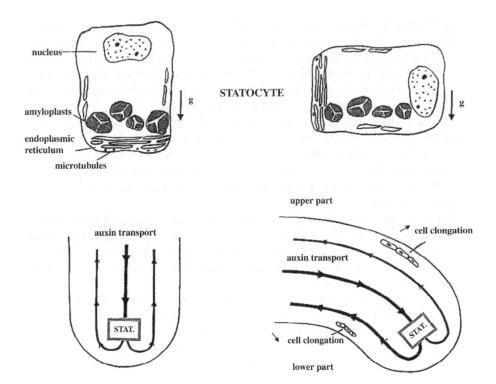

FIGURE 38 *The amyloplast response to gravity*

When amyloplasts are in their normal position (i.e., if the root is vertical), the amyloplasts are located near the basal part of the cell and induce the release of a hormone, auxin, which is equally distributed in the root.

When the root is placed in a horizontal position, the amyloplasts move towards the lower side of the cell. As a result a large fraction of the hormone is concentrated to one side of the root where cell division and elongation are slowed down (auxin has an inhibitory effect). On the other hand, cell division and, especially, elongation are stimulated in the upper half of the root. These changes in auxin distribution are responsible for root bending (root gravitropism). (From Planel, H. *L' Espace et la Vie.* Larousse, Paris, 1988.)

being localized toward the superior or proximal pole of the cell while numerous endoplasmic reticulum lacunae occupy the distal pole. These cells are essentially characterized by the presence of large granules called amyloplasts since they mostly contain starch. On Earth and in a vertical growing position, amyloplasts occupy the bottom half of the cell (Figure 38). Owing to their weight, they exert pressure or traction on the microtubules or fibrils of the cytoskeleton close to them. This induces the release of a hormone called auxin, thereby transforming the gravity signal into a chemically mediated signal. Later, auxin, diffuses in the surrounding cells, which are themselves stimulated by growth-stimulating hormones. Unlike the latter, auxin has an inhibitory action, at least on the root. Under normal growth conditions, auxin diffuses in a regular fashion in all cells, which explains the vertical orientation of the root.

Supposing the root is placed in the horizontal position, the amyloplasts are now going to slide toward the lower lateral wall of the statocytes. Auxin, under these conditions, will direct itself more particularly toward neighboring cells occupying the lower side of the root. This novel distribution can be observed with various techniques and, in particular, using radioactive auxin as shown in the experiments of Mariko Oka and co-workers at the University of Osaka.

Auxin is, therefore, transported asymmetrically when the root is placed in a horizontal position, and this phenomenon is the origin of the geotropic response. Indeed, cellular growth will be inhibited in the bottom half of the root where auxin is concentrated. Growth, on the other hand, will be stimulated in the top half, and the differential growth will provoke the curvature of the root characteristic of the geotropic response.

Does this mean that the gravitropic curving response is the result of an increase in cellular division in the upper half of the root? The hypothesis can be rejected on the grounds that root cells divide every 25 hours, whereas the gravitropic response occurs within 2 hours. Growth changes are, in fact, due to an increase in cell volume (otherwise called elongation).

Auxin does not act alone. Indeed the endoplasmic reticulum releases calcium, which is immediately fixed by a special protein known as calmodulin. The calmodulin-calcium complex migrates toward enzymes located in the membrane of statocytes and acting as calcium or auxin pumps. Once activated, they allow the calcium and calmodulin hormone to exit and diffuse toward neighboring cells (Figure 39).

Amyloplasts in the root cap play an essential role—comparable to that of otoliths in the vestibular apparatus—in the gravitropic reaction mechanism. Nevertheless, as nothing is ever simple in biology, the geotropic response can still be observed in an *Arabidopsis thaliana* mutant in which the cells have no amyloplasts. Fortunately, however, this exception is readily explained. In this case, nucleus migration substitutes for amyloplast displacement, thereby provoking a geotropic response. The latter is, however, more discrete than in the wild type.

Though the behavior of this mutant can be explained, many questions still remain unresolved. For instance, the molecular mechanism of geotropism is still obscure. It would, therefore, be madness not to take advantage of the extraordinary tool that space research represents since it is the only means of exposing plants to genuine microgravity.

EFFECTS OF WEIGHTLESSNESS

Since the beginning of space research, a fairly large number of experiments have been conducted, whether on developing seeds or plantules. Germinating wheat seeds as well as onion bulbs were able to develop in space. On several occasions, stimulation phenomena were even observed by Russian scientists. In addition, present knowledge about the geotropic response suggested that plant morphology might be modified in space. This hypothesis was confirmed many years ago now with pepper plants onboard the American Biosatellite-2. Although the flight only lasted 48 hours, a rapid disorientation of the stem and leaves was found. It is of interest to note that

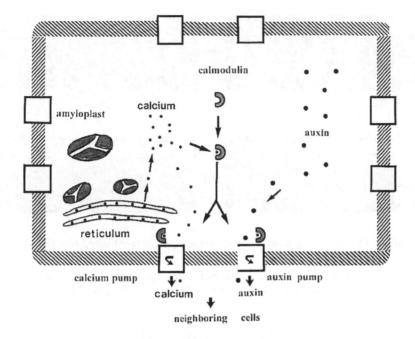

FIGURE 39 *The mechanism of gravitropism*

The gravitropic response is induced by calcium ions released from the endoplasmic reticulum vesicles. The Ca⁺⁺ ions are fixed by the protein, calmodulin. This complex can then activate enzymes in the membrane acting as auxin pumps and calcium channels. However, many steps in this mechanism are still under discussion. (From Planel, H. *L' Espace et la Vie*. Larousse, Paris, 1988.)

this response as well as certain biochemical modifications lasted longer than those induced on the ground by clinostat experimentation over the same length of time.

Another question was raised: can a plant grow normally in the absence of gravity? This question is not only important from the point of view of fundamental biology but also for its practical repercussions since the culture of certain plants has been envisaged on space stations. The answer to this question was given thanks to *Arabidopsis*, a plant offering the dual advantage of being small, less than 20 cm in height, and having a life cycle of a mere few weeks.

Seeds were therefore made to germinate onboard Salyut-7 in an area endowed with a lighting apparatus and continuous air supply. The results turned out spectacular; the seeds developed well and gave rise to plants that flowered and produced seeds. When studied later, these seeds were themselves fertile and capable of germination. Thus, an entire life cycle had occurred in spite of the absence of gravity. Microgravity, however, did bring about certain changes: slower growth and lower numbers of leaves per rosette than normal. Furthermore, while the total length of the plants was 17.5 cm in the controls, the length of the plants cultivated on Salyut-7 was only 9.6 cm. Finally, the seeds were smaller than normal. These facts confirm

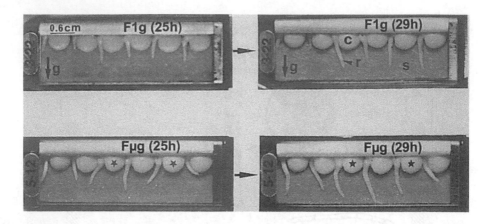

FIGURE 40 *The response of lentil seedlings to microgravity (see Color figure VIII at the end of the book)*

In space, the emerging roots are bent under microgravity but remain in a vertical position, as on Earth, when placed in a 1 *g* centrifuge (Pr. G. Perbal, University of Paris).

that gravity does not only affect plant orientation, but also, in this particular case, growth and morphology. Care must be taken not to jump to conclusions, however, since growth in other species seems to be normal and development barely altered (Figure 40).

Studies have also been undertaken in the Biorack program onboard the Challenger Shuttle. The disorientation of roots from germinating seeds was again observed. G. Perbal, from the University Pierre et Marie Curie, has also shown that statocytes from lentil plantules having differentiated and developed under microgravity conditions were still capable of reacting to a given acceleration, in this case a 1 *g* centrifuge used onboard the shuttle (Figure 40). The influence of gravity on amyloplasts was also confirmed in lentils and watercress plantules where microgravity did provoke their dispersion within the statocytes. Instead of being concentrated toward the lower side of these cells, the amyloplasts were spread throughout the cytoplasm (Figure 41). This clearly demonstrates that amyloplasts are the gravity-sensing organelles of plants. Interestingly, scientists from the University of Colorado working on clover have shown that while amyloplasts are put, as it were, at rest under microgravity conditions, they are still able to differentiate and synthesize starch in developing plantules.

Perbal and co-workers calculated the presentation time for lentil plantules in the Spacelab during the IML-1 shuttle mission. The method is certainly simpler than it is on Earth. The presentation time is obtained by placing the plantules previously developed under microgravity on a small 1 *g* centrifuge and then returning them to microgravity. When this is done, a modification of the initial curvature reflects the appearance of a gravitropic response. These results remarkably confirm the observations made in previous experiments: the presentation time is indeed on the order of 27 seconds only.

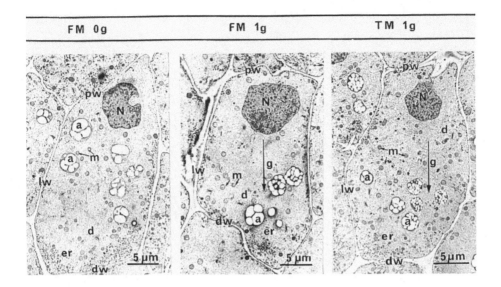

FIGURE 41 *The effects of microgravity on statocyte structure (electron micrograph)*

Under microgravity (FM 0 g), the nucleus tends to move away from the cell membrane, and the amyloplasts are distributed throughout the cell. When lentil seeds are placed in a 1 g centrifuge aboard the shuttle (FM 1 *g*), the microgravity effects disappear. The control (TM 1 *g*) was carried out on Earth (Pr. G. Perbal, University of Paris). Similar results were obtained in clinostat experiments on Earth.

Finally, electronic microscope studies of lentil plantules have shown that the statocyte skeleton plays a role in the gravitropic response. As already mentioned in the chapter on cellular biology, it is likely that the long-ignored relationship between gravity and the various elements of the cytoskeleton will slowly be elucidated, space research providing a significant input in the resolution of this issue.

12 Developmental Biology

The question has been raised whether living organisms can reproduce in space. In other words, are mating, fertilization, embryonic development and delivery possible in the absence of gravity? This is important because humans may one day undertake long-term space missions. These questions are not easily answered though it has been known for some time that certain species can reproduce in microgravity. This was true of Drosophila fruit flies used in genetic experiments aboard the first satellites. Later, the Spanish biologist R. Marco observed during a Spacelab mission that although oocyte production was normal, there were less embryos and larvae hatching and developing from these oocytes. Other experiments performed aboard Skylab-3 and on the Apollo-Soyuz mission showed that fish eggs from Fundulus killifish developed with important abnormalities in different systems or organs like the cardiovascular and visual systems, and the vestibular apparatus. However, any gravity-induced effects are likely to go undetected since they would only occur during the first steps of embryonic development before compensatory mechanisms came into play to regulate them. In other words, no answers can be given without having the biological material and equipment necessary for studying the influence of gravity on fertilization and the first steps of egg and embryo development. New space experiments have been performed with this objective on amphibians, sea urchins and fish eggs.

AMPHIBIAN EGGS

Amphibian eggs[1] such as frog eggs are polarized, that is, the structure of the upper or animal pole differs from that of the lower or vegetal pole (Figure 42). The animal pole contains large amounts of melanin, a black pigment identical to the one found in skin. Melanin is concentrated in the superficial part or cortex of the oocyte, the mature germ cell produced in the ovary. Most of the volume of the oocyte is occupied by yolk platelets, which are concentrated in the vegetal pole. This part of the germ cell lacks pigment granules. When oocytes are laid, they are surrounded by a vitelline membrane and wrapped in a jelly mass. After having been laid in fresh water, oocytes are randomly oriented with respect to gravity. Once the sperm penetrates the oocyte and fertilization takes place, the cortex shrinks and separates from the vitelline membrane. The egg subsequently rotates so that the lighter animal pole is oriented upward and the heavy vegetal pole downward, thus demonstrating the influence of gravity. Important structural changes occur shortly afterward when the cortex rotates

---

[1] Before fertilization, it is more correct to use the term "oocyte." After fertilization, the term egg is still widely used since the first cellular divisions occur without volume modification.

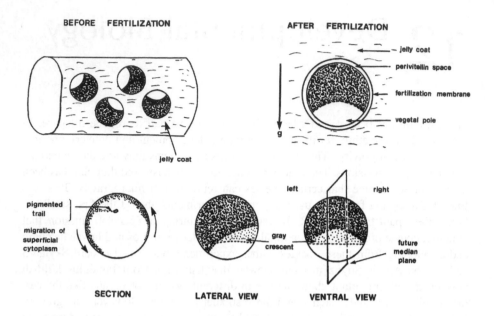

FIGURE 42 *Gravity and amphibian egg development*

The eggs of amphibians are wrapped in a gelatinous mass. They contain a black pigment and are randomly oriented with respect to gravity.

After fertilization, the egg rotates and the pigment is located in the upper part of the egg. A rotation of the peripheral part or cortex reveals a less pigmented zone, the gray crescent. The plane that crosses the middle of the gray crescent corresponds to the plane of the first egg division and indicates the bilateral plane of symmetry of the embryo.

with respect to the rest of the cytoplasm. Whereas the boundary between the pigmented and nonpigmented zones of the oocyte was nearly horizontal, the 15 to 30° rotation now causes it to become oblique. The downward movement of the boundary reveals a less pigmented zone on the opposite side known as the gray crescent. Sperm is involved in these changes since the penetration point of the male gamete in the oocyte orients the movement of the cortex. Indeed, the sliding movement of the cortex occurs on the side where the sperm penetrates the oocyte.

The cytoskeleton plays an important role in these structural changes of the egg in that they involve a sliding of microtubules and a contraction of actin filaments.

The changes just described reflect a novel polarization of the egg. The plane that crosses the middle of the gray crescent corresponds to the bilateral symmetry plane, and the two egg halves on either side of it will give rise to the left and right parts of the embryo. The gray crescent also corresponds to the dorsal side of the future embryo where the small circular opening called the blastopore eventually appears (Figure 43). The outer cells of the embryo, called blastula, invaginate and give rise to a germ cell layer called chordomesoderm. The cells move deep inside the embryo, which becomes a gastrula. After gastrulation, the embryo consists of three germ layers: (1) ectoderm which covers the embryo and will form the skin and nervous system, (2) endoderm which is the primordium of the digestive tract, and (3) chordomesoderm which gives rise to many tissues such as connective, muscle and bone tissue.

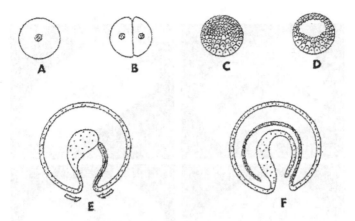

FIGURE 43 *The first stages of embryonic development in amphibians*

A: Fertilized egg

B: Stage II: 2-cell stage (two embryonic cells called blastomeres)

C: Morula

D: Blastula with a cavity or blastocoele

E: Gastrula. Invagination of the superficial embryonic cells at the blastopore site.

F: End of gastrula. There is an innermost layer or endoderm and an outermost layer or ectoderm. Between the two lies the mesoderm.

Experiments carried out on Earth suggest that gravity plays a role in the first steps of amphibian egg development. For instance, if an egg is maintained in an inverted position after fertilization or placed in a slow clinostat, the gravity-induced effects on the different parts of the egg are modified and frequent changes in gray crescent and blastopore localization are noted. However, regulatory phenomena later lead to normal development.

Does space research confirm the influence of gravity on embryogenesis? The first space experiments showed that fertilization can occur in weightlessness as was demonstrated on rocket flights using oocytes from Xenopus, a frog often used in the laboratory. Only one sperm fertilized the oocyte, as happens on Earth, and the cortical reactions that block penetration by other sperms continued normally in microgravity. A complex experimental device used during the IML-1 mission showed that Xenopus oocytes fertilized in space developed normally up to the gastrula stage before their return to Earth. Later, G. A. Ubbels of Utrecht in the Netherlands confirmed these results by injecting females on a space flight with gonadotrophic hormone to induce ovulation. The oocytes were placed with sperm that had been conserved *in vitro*. After fertilization, the embryos gave birth to tadpoles that swam as well as those born on Earth. Another experiment carried out during the IML-2 mission showed embryonic cell division was not modified in weightlessness.

The question then is whether it is possible to conclude from these results that gravity is not essential for establishing the dorsal-ventral symmetry plane in Xenopus. This appears to be the case when taking into account K. Souza's experiment carried out aboard the Shuttle. *In vitro* kept sperm was used to fertilize Xenopus oocytes produced in space after injecting hormones into females. Although a few abnormalities were observed in the embryos arrested in the gastrula stage, the experiment

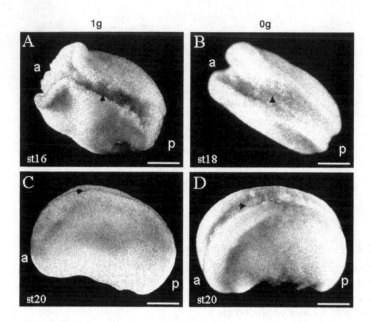

FIGURE 44 *The Pleurodel experiment*
This experiment was carried out aboard the Mir space station. Eggs from the amphibian Pleurodel fertilized in orbit were able to develop. However, certain abnormalities were observed, particularly in the nervous system formation. The picture shows the abnormal development of the medullar groove, which gives rise to the central nervous system (Lydie Parisot *et al.* experiment).

showed that development carried on normally. Still more recently Anne-Marie Duprat *et al.* carried out another experiment on salamander (Pleurodel) during the French-Russian Cassiopia mission aboard Mir (Figure 44). The females, which had already mated and were carrying sperm stored in vesicles connected to the genital ducts, were injected during the flight with pituitary hormone to induce oocyte production. Embryonic development led to normal tadpoles, but films and post-flight studies showed that the embryonic cells had a tendency to pull away from one another. The small protuberances or microvilli on the surface of the egg were also less developed than normal. In some cases the closing of the medullar groove looked altered.

These results tend to show that gravity can affect the first steps of embryonic development and suggest that the effects of microgravity are compensated by regulatory phenomena. Perhaps microgravity also alters certain cells that are expelled, with the remaining cells ensuring embryonic development. Nevertheless, this research shows once again the usefulness of space studies, without which gravity would still be considered essential for the embryonic development of amphibian eggs and the establishment of the bilateral symmetry plane of the embryo and future organism.

SEA URCHIN AND FISH EGGS

Sea urchin fertilization occurs in the environmental medium and can easily be carried out *in vitro*, making it suitable material for study. Furthermore, since fertilization is short it can take place on rocket probe flights. Hans-Jürg Marthy carried out several experiments and found in each case that fertilization and the resulting structural changes in the egg occurred normally. Kenichi Ijiri of Tokyo, Japan broke more ground when he studied whether mating was possible in microgravity. He investigated the behavior of *Orizias latipes* or Madaka killifish. In these small freshwater fish, fertilization occurs during mating and the females lay eggs that develop soon afterward. Two males and two females on the IML-2 mission in 1994 were observed and photographed two, four and seven days after launch. The experiment showed that mating, egg laying and embryonic development occurred normally. The baby fish born in space swam normally even after recovery, whereas the parents, who had lost the use of their air bladder under weightlessness and remained at the bottom of the aquarium, only resumed normal swimming four days after recovery. The doors of space aquaculture were thus opened.

MAMMALS

It is easy to understand why we still have very little data on mammals. One experiment showed that the histological structure of the testicles of rats flown aboard Cosmos-1167 was not modified. Their sexual behavior did not change after recovery, and there was no decrease in the sperm fertilization capacity. Another experiment carried out aboard Cosmos-1167 using females in the second stage of gestation showed that delivery occurred normally after recovery. It is too early to ascertain whether weightlessness affected embryonic development and the formation of certain organs. However, posture reflex modifications were noted in young rats shortly after their birth. The responses to physiological tests could be explained by a late development of the vestibular apparatus during the space flight. On Earth, the gestation pattern of guinea pigs exposed to 1.3 to 2 *g* on Earth was not modified, but the number of living neonates was greater than normal. In rats, opposite results were reported.

As for humans, the issue of reproduction has often been raised. Although mixed crews have been asked off-color questions, nothing has admittedly transpired so far. However, fertilization should be possible because astronauts are capable of having erections, and the long migration of spermatozoa in the female genital ducts seems to be gravity independent.

EVOLUTION AND GRAVITY

While a possible influence of gravity on the embryonic development of living organisms, i.e., on ontogeny, has to date not been demonstrated, it is obvious that gravity has played a major role on the evolution of species, i.e., on phylogeny. A great number of arguments plead in favor of this notion and show the value of space research in this particular area of developmental biology. Atmospheric composition and volcanic activity have acted upon each other, with the occurrence of cold and warm eras, while ground radioactivity gradually decreased. However, gravity being directly linked to the Earth's mass is the only environmental factor that has remained unchanged since the formation of the planet and the first appearance of living organisms. Thus all living beings have always been exposed to the influence of gravity, making it a major factor in the evolution of species.

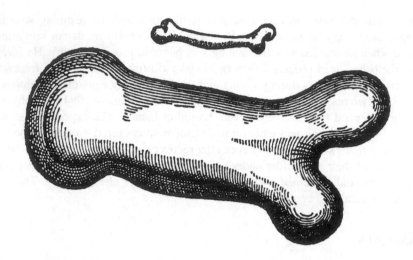

FIGURE 45 *Gravity and evolution*

As early as 1538, Galileo noted that the bones of large animals are thicker than the bones of small creatures. This is quite logical since volume and weight vary as a function of the cube of body length.

In good agreement with this idea, the skeleton, muscles, the cardiovascular and other systems are proof of an adaptation to gravity. Galileo first pointed out such an influence in 1538 after studying the skeleton of various mammals (Figure 45). He observed that the bones supporting the weight of the body were proportionally thicker in taller species than in shorter ones, a logical state of affairs since volume and weight vary as a function of the cube of body length. The skeleton of a shrew weighs only 5 g and corresponds to 5% of its total body weight, while the skeleton of an elephant represents 35% of its total weight.

The morphology and physiology of various organisms demonstrate the influence of gravity. In humans, for instance, the great number of vein valves in the lower limb struggle against gravity-induced blood flow. In giraffes, whose height constitutes a real challenge to gravity, blood pressure near the heart is double that of humans and allows the blood to reach the brain situated 1.20 m higher. In birds, the bones are less dense and have a system of cavities that make them lighter than the bones of terrestrial species. This facilitates flight and decreases energy loss. Gravity effects are also demonstrated when comparing terrestrial and aquatic species. In the latter, the influence of gravity is less significant since it is partly compensated for by the Archimedes push. The skeleton of aquatic vertebrates is less developed and represents, for example, only 15% of the total body weight of the whale.

The size and shape of certain bones also differ according to lifestyle. In very large mammals like the elephant and the rhinoceros, the spine and rib cage stretch to allow a better distribution of visceral pressure, a particularity that is less obvious in the hippopotamus, which lives both on land and in water. In very small species, factors linked to the aquatic environment have acted in association with gravity during evolution. An example of this is surface tension, which is the force that tends to make liquids rise up the edges of a container. With this in mind, D'Arcy Thomson carried out the following curious experiment: he let a drop of viscous liquid fall into a more fluid environment where it moved easily under the effect of gravity. However, since the surface tension forces slowed down its course, it broke into numerous fragments to form something that looked like a jellyfish. The weaker influence of gravity also explains the highly complex shape of certain aquatic species such as plankton, which have long appendages that species living on the ground could not carry or move. However, aquatic species are not sheltered from gravitational effects as the frequent changes in swimming orientation create sudden accelerations. It can be assumed that the first vertebrates that left the water environment to lead a terrestrial life had already partly adapted to gravity.

In summary, gravity has been a factor in the evolution of animal and plant species, which explains the importance of studying the behavior patterns of carefully selected species with short life cycles, such as Drosophila fruit flies, over successive generations in space. It should be of great interest to know if changes in gravitational force bring DNA modifications resulting in changes in embryonic development and features of certain species.

13 Cosmic Radiation

Cosmic radiation, like gravity, exists at all points on the planet. It does not affect sensory organs the way light does and most people are unaware of its existence. What is this mysterious radiation from space and what are its effects, especially on manned missions in space?

A FEW CONCEPTS IN PHYSICS

THE DISCOVERY OF COSMIC RADIATION

Take a small gas-filled vessel with two metallic plates by way of electrodes. Link the electrodes to the two terminals of a battery: nothing happens. Now, if you expose the gas to ionizing radiation, the gas molecules lose or gain electrons to become ions that are then displaced toward one electrode or the other depending upon their electric charge. An electric current thus passes between the metallic plates, and its magnitude indicates the level of ionization and the intensity of the radiation.

A young Austrian physicist named Victor Hess made a fundamental discovery when using a similar ionization chamber, a precursor of today's Geiger counter. Hess was a remarkable mountain climber, as were all his colleagues studying cosmic radiation during that period. While climbing the alpine summits in the early 1910s, he observed that the natural ionizing radiation increased with altitude.

Hess found further support for his theory on July 7, 1912 when, after several attempts, he rose to an altitude of 4500 m in an air balloon. He first observed a decrease in the radiation level compared to that measured on the ground, but then noted that the radiation intensity increased as the balloon gained altitude. He understood that this radiation, invisible to the naked eye but detectable by special instruments, must originate from space and was for the most part absorbed by the Earth's atmosphere. In 1936, he received the Nobel Prize for his work in physics.

The introduction of stratospheric balloons, rocket probes and especially spacecraft technology have allowed us to increase our understanding of the nature and origin of cosmic rays and their biological effects. Indeed, although considered harmless up to that point, cosmic rays were found to have biological effects that could potentially pose a serious risk to human beings in space. Due to the fact that cosmic radiation is very complex in composition, the risks are difficult to evaluate using classical radiation biology data.

COMPOSITION OF COSMIC RADIATION

In space, humans are exposed to three types of radiation: solar wind, galactic cosmic rays and radiation belts. The first two make up cosmic radiation (Figure 46).

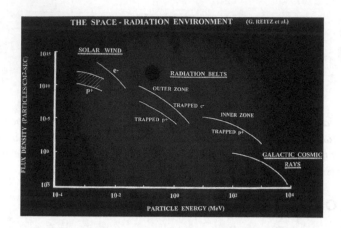

FIGURE 46 *Radiation in space*

Man in space is exposed to three types of radiation: solar wind made of protons and electrons, radiation belts made of particles trapped by the magnetic field of the Earth and galactic rays made of very high energy particles originating from star explosions (redrawn from G. Reitz).

Solar Wind

In addition to visible light, the sun emits ultraviolet and infrared radiation. It also emits another kind of radiation called solar wind. Solar wind is complex in nature, comprising ionizing electromagnetic radiation, in particular X-rays and gamma rays. These are made up of X- or gamma photons, which have more energy than the photons of visible light. Solar wind also contains electrons and protons (i.e., hydrogen nuclei) that are constantly emitted by the sun. Most of these particles are low-energy particles, on the order of a few keV (kiloelectron-volts), and move at a speed of approximately 400 km per second.

In addition to solar wind, the sun emits other kinds of radiation during solar flares, which will be discussed below.

Galactic Cosmic Rays

Galactic rays result from the explosion of certain stars. All stars, including the sun, burn their constituents in a series of nuclear explosions, thus using up their fuel little by little. At the end of their evolution very large stars—but not the sun since it is only a medium-sized star—cool down, contract and become incredibly dense. Once they reach the final phase, they explode, become supernovae and eject a multitude of particles in space. The formation of a supernova is a very rare phenomenon and is only seldom witnessed. One was seen in the Taurus constellation on July 4, 1054 and another was observed in the Cassiopeia constellation in 1572. Tycho Brahe, a Dane who made remarkable discoveries even without an astronomical telescope, was one of its witnesses. In 1604, numerous astronomers including Johannes Kepler identified another supernova. Since then, thanks to new astronomical instruments, other supernovae have been detected, and it is estimated that two or three occur per century in galaxies similar to ours. One of the most recent supernovae was detected as soon as it began to form in the Great Magellan cloud on February 23, 1987.

Although it is known that the explosion of a supernova gives rise to galactic rays, the precise origin of this type of radiation remains poorly understood. A possible source is a supernova dating from 1006 AD, which is believed to have appeared as bright as the moon for several centuries. There are other probable sources, but they are extremely difficult to detect. The magnetic and electric fields of the different stars in the galaxy deflect the particles emitted by supernova remnants. The particles are subject to successive reflections and their exact point of origin cannot be ascertained. During their long journey toward Earth, these particles are progressively accelerated and acquire a lot of energy, which varies from 100 to 1000 MeV (millions of electron volts) or more. Some may even have more energy than that obtained in the largest accelerators.

Galactic cosmic rays, like solar wind, are complex in nature. They are made up of protons (87%), alpha particles or helium nuclei (12%) and heavy ions (1%). The latter particles, sometimes referred to as HZE particles (high Z and high energy particles), correspond to the nuclei of atoms with an atomic number Z (the number of positive charges in the nucleus) greater than 2. Despite their relative scarcity, these particles are of major biological importance.

Radiation Belts

Astrophysicists predicted the existence of radiation belts well before their discovery. In 1985, the American physicist James Van Allen found the first evidence that confirmed this theory during the flight of Explorer-1, the first American satellite. This marked one of the first contributions of space-based research to astrophysics. The Van Allen belts are the result of the interaction of cosmic rays and the terrestrial magnetic field. William Gilbert, an English medical doctor of the early 17th century, demonstrated that the Earth was a magnet. Sailors had been navigating using compasses based on this principle for over a thousand years before Gilbert's discovery. The Earth is thus surrounded by a magnetic field, occupying a zone referred to as the magnetosphere. The terrestrial magnetic field is created by the presence of iron in the central core of our planet. The lines of force of this magnetic field converge toward the two magnetic poles, which do not exactly coincide with the geographic North and South Poles.

As they approach the Earth, the solar wind and galactic cosmic rays hit the terrestrial magnetic field (Figure 47). The particles in solar wind, and to a lesser extent those in galactic cosmic rays, are first deflected by the terrestrial magnetic field on the side of the Earth facing the sun, or day side. They then penetrate the magnetosphere on the side opposite to the sun, or night side. Galactic ray particles are also directed toward the polar regions and interact with the nuclei of terrestrial atmosphere molecules. The neutrons, which are released, decay into protons and electrons that also get trapped by the magnetic field. Other high-energy particles of galactic origin may penetrate the magnetosphere and approach the Earth.

In this way, the terrestrial magnetic field traps many cosmic radiation particles, which accumulate as the two Van Allen belts. The inner belt is approximately 3,500 km above the Earth, and the outer belt lies farther away at an altitude of 20,000 km. The inner belt consists of electrons and protons while the external belt contains only electrons. Because the barriers between the two are not clearly defined, they are often simply referred to jointly as the radiation belt. The trapped particles are in perpetual motion, and their flux can reach several millions per cm^2 per second.

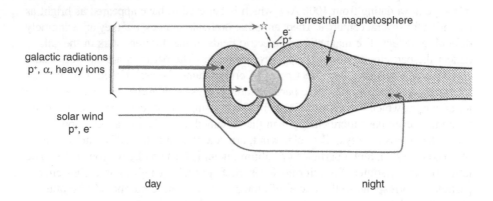

FIGURE 47 *Cosmic rays and the magnetic field of the Earth (see Color figure IX at the end of the book)*

Solar wind low-energy particles are deflected by the Earth's magnetic field on the day side but can penetrate on the night side where the Earth's magnetic field is weaker. Some particles of galactic radiation reach the polar region. High-energy particles can cross the Earth's magnetic field but most are trapped by it, giving rise to radiation belts.

Based on these figures, the belts should not present a threat for manned flights, which generally take place at altitudes of only 300 to 400 km. However, satellite studies have shown that the innermost belt can extend down to the Earth's surface. In the Southern Hemisphere, off the Brazilian and Argentinean coasts, the belt is only 160 to 320 km above the surface of the planet and can sometimes even descend into the upper layers of the atmosphere. This particular region is known as the South Atlantic Anomaly (SAA) and its origin is unknown. It might be the result of a discontinuity, a hole in the terrestrial magnetic field. It could also be due to the displacement between the geographical and geomagnetic centers of the Earth, which would bring the inner belt closer to the South American coast and farther away from the Earth in diametrically opposed regions.

PRIMARY AND SECONDARY COSMIC RADIATION

Taken together, solar and galactic cosmic radiation is known as primary cosmic radiation. In practice, the crew in a spacecraft is exposed to secondary cosmic radiation. While the walls of a spacecraft stop most primary cosmic radiation particles, some can penetrate the wall material. The resulting interactions yield secondary particles of the same nature as primary particles but weaker in energy, as well as neutrons and X-rays. These types of radiation constitute secondary cosmic radiation.

On the ground, living organisms are also exposed to secondary cosmic radiation in part made up of particles that have penetrated the barrier of the magnetic field. On the other hand, while certain protons do reach the surface of the Earth, most of the primary cosmic radiation is stopped by the terrestrial atmosphere (Figure 48). Alpha particles and heavy ions practically disappear at an altitude of 20,000 m, but protons

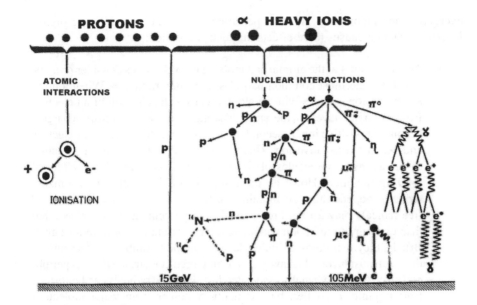

FIGURE 48 *Primary and secondary cosmic rays*

In free space, every object is exposed to primary cosmic radiation. Inside a spacecraft or at the Earth's surface, men are exposed to secondary cosmic radiation.
Near the Earth, most cosmic radiation particles collide with the nuclei of atmospheric atoms, giving out electromagnetic radiation and various particles. Natural ionizing radiation or background radiation consists of the secondary cosmic radiation as well as ground radioactivity.

are able to penetrate deeper. All of these particles collide with the oxygen and nitrogen atoms of the atmosphere. As a result, these atoms lose electrons and the air gets ionized, a phenomenon possibly responsible for stimulatory or harmful effects. In fact, most collisions occur with the nuclei of atmospheric atoms and the resulting interactions give rise to electromagnetic radiation, in particular gamma rays and various particles such as electrons, neutrons and mesons. Some of these particles, neutrinos for instance, are able to cross the Earth. This radiation constitutes secondary cosmic radiation on the surface of the Earth. Natural ionizing radiation or background radiation consists of this secondary cosmic radiation as well as ground radioactivity.

Due to its extensive energy spectrum and heterogeneous composition, cosmic radiation is difficult to reproduce on the ground. Accelerators can only generate radiation of a fixed nature and energy. This difficulty is enhanced, as cosmic radiation and weightlessness may have combined effects. Simulation of these two factors is currently impossible technologically.

RADIATION BIOLOGY: GENERAL CONCEPTS

THE EFFECTS OF IONIZING RADIATION

Like the X-rays or gamma rays of cobalt bombs, cosmic radiation is an ionizing radiation. (Direct or indirect ionizing radiation will not be addressed in this book). In this sense, it is different from ultraviolet and infrared radiation, which are less energetic and nonionizing. When it penetrates inert matter or a living organism, ionizing radiation causes three effects in quick succession:

- The first occurs at the atomic and molecular level. Let us consider protons, which are the most common particles in cosmic radiation. When a high-energy proton collides with an atom, it causes the ejection of an electron from the outer layer of the atom. The atom, initially neutrally charged, becomes a positive ion. A second atom can then catch the ejected electron and become a negative ion. This proton has thus modified the structure of the atoms or molecules of living matter. This is the direct effect of ionizing radiation. However, the responses of living matter to ionizing radiation depend more on an indirect effect, in which the much-discussed free radicals play a role. Free radicals can be generated by means other than exposure to radiation and are to a large extent responsible for aging. Briefly, they are atoms or molecules with an odd number of electrons, in the outermost layer. This layer has an "unpaired" electron, whereas peripheral electrons are normally associated in pairs. Free radicals can be formed from organic molecules, but the majority comes from water molecules (H_2O), which split after several steps into two free radicals, $H^{\bullet}$ and $OH^{\bullet}$. This occurs at a surprising rate: an ionizing water molecule dissociates in less than 10^{-11} seconds. The free radicals, which diffuse very rapidly, are extremely reactive. Because of their oxidizing power (for $OH^{\bullet}$) or reducing power (for $H^{\bullet}$), they can attack neighboring organic molecules. Despite their extremely short life span, they can produce important structural changes in the molecules of living matter.

  All molecules can be modified by the direct or indirect action of radiation, but irradiation has the most impact on molecules that play a fundamental role in the life of the cell. Enzymatic proteins that control metabolism and DNA[1], which controls the synthesis of proteins, are particularly at risk.
- The second effect of ionizing radiation occurs at the cellular level. Ionizing radiation, which induces modifications at the molecular level, can affect the functions of a cell and even lead to its death. Some responses occur rapidly, within several hours after exposure to radiation, while others develop over a longer period of time. Much of the damage done affects DNA molecules; this includes single- and double-strand breaks, base modifications and base mispairing. Some of this damage can be repaired, but structural changes that are inadequately repaired or allowed to persist can often lead to modifications in chromosome morphology. Modifications at the gene level are responsible for mutations. DNA damage can persist for many years in the ovaries and testicles of irradiated individuals. If sex cells, sperm and ovum, have altered DNA, the damage can be transmitted to the offspring.

---

[1] The two strands of a DNA molecule are complementary in their nucleotide sequences and paired in a double helix. Each nucleotide contains a molecule of phosphoric acid, a molecule of sugar and a base (adenine linked to thymine, cytosine linked to guanine in the complementary strand).

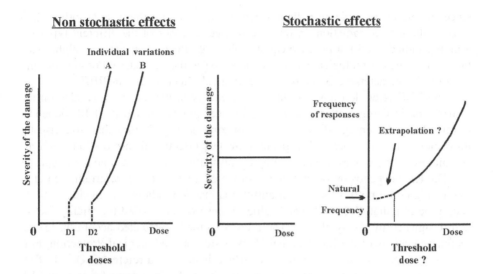

FIGURE 49 *Response to ionizing radiation*

In the case of nonstochastic effects such as skin burns or redness (left), the damage depends, above a certain threshold and for all individuals, on the dose and nature of the radiation. For stochastic effects (right) the response only occurs, for the same dose, in some individuals. The nature and the amplitude of the response are always the same but, in this case, it is the probability of occurrence that depends on the dose. Radiation-induced cancer is, for instance, a stochastic radiation effect.

• Finally, cellular damage may create problems at the organ and whole organism level. Responses that appear systematically, regardless of the individual, are called nonstochastic effects (Figure 49). In this case, above a certain threshold, the extent of radiation-induced sickness depends on the dose and nature of radiation exposure (single, repeated, chronic, partial or whole body irradiation). Cataracts, skin redness or burns, damage to bone marrow and the intestinal mucous membrane are all nonstochastic effects.

Stochastic effects, on the other hand, are those which are generated only in some individuals. The nature and amplitude of the responses are always the same, but the probability of their appearance depends on the dose received, as in the case of cancer. An injury either initiates cancer or it does not. Nonstochastic effects appear most often within several hours or several days after irradiation while stochastic effects may take many years to develop.

Doses in Radiation Biology and Their Meaning

Cosmic radiation loses its energy when it penetrates living matter. The energy thus transferred to the living system is classically expressed in rads, a rad corresponding to 100 ergs absorbed by 1 g of matter. The gray is the more commonly used unit (1 gray = 100 rads). In biology and medicine, dose equivalents are more often used since the effects of ionizing radiation depend, not only on the dose absorbed, but also on the type of radiation. In other words, equal doses of the different types of ionizing radiation do not produce equal biological effects. For instance, alpha particles cause greater biological damage than X-rays at the same dose. For this reason, each ray is characterized by its relative biological effectiveness, or RBE.

The RBE value depends not only on the energy of the radiation but also on its distribution in living matter. Energy loss induces ionization and the RBE depends ultimately on the energy distribution or ionizing density. X-rays that give rise to ionization events that are well separated are less effective than radiation, such as cosmic rays, which gives rise to ionizing events that are very close together in space.

The RBE depends on other factors (single or fractionated dose, irradiation at a low or high dose rate). It is this variability that has led radiologists to characterize each type of radiation by a "mean" value of these factors, called the quality factor and designated by the symbol Q. The quality factor is calculated according to the recommendations of the International Commission on Radiological Protection. For X-rays and gamma radiation from ^{60}Co, which is used as a reference, Q = 1. The quality factor is greater for particle radiation; it can be 2 or more for protons, 10 for fast neutrons and 20 for alpha particles. Thus, 1 Gy of a particular radiation with a Q = 2 has the same effectiveness as 2 Gy of X-rays or gamma rays.

In conclusion, the quality factor explains that in order to obtain a better estimate of radiation damage, we must determine the dose-equivalent (expressed in rem) calculated from the absorbed dose (expressed in rads) multiplied by the quality factor Q (or QF)

$$\text{Dose-equivalent (rem)} = \text{Absorbed dose (rad)} \times Q$$

Today, the absorbed dose is expressed in grays and the dose-equivalent in Sieverts (1 Sv = 100 rem). Dose-equivalents are also expressed in milliSieverts (mSv) or thousandth of a Sievert (10^{-3} Sv) as well as in microSieverts (μSv) or millionth of a Sievert (10^{-6} Sv).

It is of great interest to determine the quality factor and dose-equivalence of cosmic rays, a very complex radiation made up of different charged particles with various energies, if we wish to estimate the radiation risks involved in manned space flights.

THE DOSIMETRY OF COSMIC RADIATION

The dosimetry (dose measurement) of cosmic radiation has been performed on each manned flight since the beginning of astronautics. Early pioneers such as E. V. Benton from the United States, Y. Gregoriev and E. E. Kovalev of the Soviet Union have greatly contributed to our knowledge on cosmic radiation. Doses are measured using passive thermoluminescent detectors, which usually contain lithium fluoride. Astronauts wear these detectors as badges to monitor individual doses. Active detectors such as proportional counters are also used; and the combination of their walls and the gas they contain is equivalent to living issue. The information these detectors provide allows one to determine absorbed doses, quality factor and dose equivalence.

TABLE 1

Shuttle	Altitude (km)	Angle (degrees)	Dose mGy/d	Equiv.Dose mSv/d
STS 51	290	28.5	0.04	0.14
STS 61	594	28.5	0.15	0.23
STS 47	300	57.0	0.05	0.20
MIR				
Aragatz	400	51.5	0.32	0.62
Antares	420	51.5	0.53	1.0
Altaïr	420	51.5	0.54	0.95

Table 1 provides an example of the typical daily doses that astronauts receive on a mission. Absorbed doses are expressed in milligrays (mGy), equivalent doses in milliSieverts (mSv).

Recent data show that the mean daily dose between 1995 and 1999 was about 0.7 mSv for Shuttle flights, including the rendezvous with Mir. The average daily dose on Mir ranges between 0.45 and 0.99 mSv and is about 0.7 mSv on the ISS.

As shown in this table, there is a great variation in the daily dose rates between different missions and the following comments can be made:

As the altitude and angle of a spacecraft increase with respect to the equatorial plane, the dose rate increases as well. It is highest near the polar regions, which explains why the doses aboard the Mir station are higher than on most manned Shuttle flights. Thus, the quality factor depends on the type of mission and its orbital characteristics. To date, Q has varied from 1.5 to 3, well above the Q = 1 for X-rays or gamma rays. For many years one of the primary objectives of space radiation biology was to determine the quality factor of cosmic radiation.

Protons of the South Atlantic anomaly contribute significantly to the magnitude of the dose. The SAA influence is remarkable considering that, in 90 minutes of orbiting, only a few minutes are spent in this region.

The dose level also depends on the nature and thickness of the spacecraft wall, which affords more or less effective protection. For the majority of manned flights, this is of the order of 3 g/cm^2,[2] but protection of the cabin itself can vary according to the equipment inside. The detectors that astronauts wear are clearly important.

Space suits used during walks or EVAs provide reduced protection, on the order of 0.5 g/cm^2. As a result the daily dose levels are greater and may reach 5 mSv or even exceed 0.1 Sv. Under such conditions the number of EVA missions that an astronaut performs during a single space flight must be limited. Generally, EVAs should be avoided as much as possible and completely over the South Atlantic anomaly.

The solar cycle also influences radiation doses and, consequently, space mission timing (Figure 50). Solar activity is estimated based on the number of sunspots. It varies over a period of approximately 11 years. Periods of minimum solar

---

[2] The value of 3 g/cm^2, divided by the density of material, itself expressed in g/cm^3, indicates the shielding thickness. For example, a shielding of 0.5 g/cm^2 is achieved by 1.85 mm of aluminum or 0.44 mm of lead.

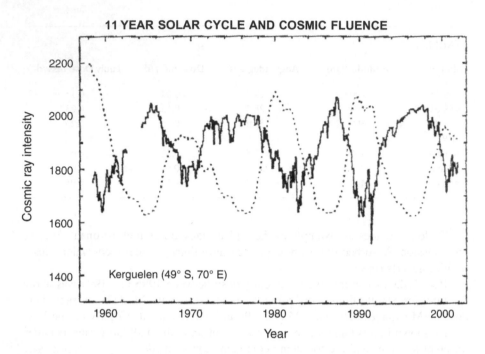

FIGURE 50 *Cosmic rays and the solar cycle*

Solar activity, estimated from the number of sunspots, varies with a periodicity of about 11 years. The intensity of cosmic radiation at the Earth's surface is linked to solar activity. (From D. Boscher.)

activity alternate with periods of maximum solar activity. This phenomenon induces cosmic radiation intensity to vary according to a cycle, the highs and lows of which are opposite to those of the solar cycle. This can easily be explained. The sun is surrounded by the planetary magnetic field. During a period of high solar activity, this magnetic field increases in such a way that its lines of force block weak-energy particles of galactic radiation traveling toward the Earth. The intensity of cosmic radiation near the Earth is thus weaker. The opposite occurs during periods of weak solar activity. However, the influence of the solar cycle is negligible for low-orbit missions because the radiation dose remains within acceptable limits.

On missions to the moon or Mars, when astronauts leave the Earth's protective magnetosphere, the radiation doses will be much greater than those on low-orbit flights. A mission between Earth and Mars would expose astronauts to a dose of about 0.25 Sv per year during a period of maximum solar activity and 0.5 Sv per year during a period of minimum solar activity. In fact, it is not easy to predict total irradiation doses: according to the adopted strategy, the mission could last between 450 and 1000 days.

Obviously, the effects of cosmic radiation are cumulative and depend on the dose received on each mission and the total number of missions in an astronaut's professional life.

THE EFFECTS OF COSMIC RADIATION

It is important to examine the extent to which radiation affects human beings in order to assess the risk in manned space flights. The risk could be important since radiation doses are greater in space than on the ground.

On Earth, it is impossible to avoid the natural ionizing radiation originating from space and ground radioactivity not to mention artificial radiation from radioactive fallout of nuclear explosions and defective nuclear reactors. The annual doses are low, on the order of 2.5 mSv; medical applications can add another 1 mSv. The dose of background radiation is greater in certain regions, such as the state of Guarapari in Brazil, Kerala in India and certain regions of China due to high levels of ground radioactivity. It is often stated that natural radiation is too weak to affect living creatures. This may be the case for humans but not for certain species, such as *Paramecium* and blue algae (Planel, H. *et al.*, 1987), since their proliferation activity may be stimulated by ground radioactivity and cosmic radiation. Regarding human beings, most of the studies on populations living in particularly radioactive sites or at high altitude have not shown an increased incidence of cancer. On the other hand, J. X. Wang found low cancer rates in Chinese populations receiving annual radiation doses three times higher than those of control populations. This effect, called hormesis, is still poorly understood. Will hormesis occur in astronauts submitted to higher levels of cosmic radiation than people on the ground? This question remains unanswered since current research focuses on the risks caused by cosmic rays.

Despite the fact that the daily radiation dose in space is approximately 20 to 100 times greater than on Earth, the radiation risk for astronauts can be considered negligible. The doses measured by global dosimetry in space are well below those capable of causing damage to the human organism. For example, during a ten-day Shuttle flight or a three-month mission aboard the Mir station, the total doses are less than 1 cSv and 10 cSv (centiSv), respectively. In the ISS, the dose for a three-month mission is about 6 cSv. In both cases these cumulative doses are the result of continuous irradiation at very low dose rate.

What are the risks of such radiation doses? A risk of nonstochastic effects arises for acute total body irradiation at much higher doses. Serious damage occurs in the bone marrow and the intestinal mucosa and is associated with bleeding and infection. A dose of 4.5 Sv leads to death within several weeks in 50% of irradiated individuals. This scenario is not a concern for low-orbit flights around the Earth but could be one when contemplating missions to other planets. Another nonstochastic risk is cataract induction. During the aging process, opacification of the lens often occurs. Cataract can also be induced by single or repeated irradiation. The latter bears some resemblance with irradiation in space but on Earth, it is necessary to reach a dose of approximately 5.5 Sv, which is much greater than the doses measured during orbital space flights.

The risks of stochastic effects, based on the total absorbed doses measured by the astronauts' badges, also appear to be low. Indeed, studies performed on the survivors of Hiroshima and Nagasaki and on other populations exposed to radiation have shown that acute exposure below 200 mSv or low dose-rate exposures below 500 mSv do not produce carcinogenic effects. Astronauts may still be at risk since they are exposed to low doses and the need for further information on the effects of such doses on the incidence of cancer is clear. Furthermore, there could be a threshold or minimum dose above which carcinogenic effects are observed. In spite of these uncertainties, it can be assumed that astronauts' exposure to cosmic rays can increase the risk of excess fatal cancer by 3%, the same as that experienced by radiation workers on Earth.

Cosmic radiation may also produce genetic damage, another stochastic effect. Many years ago, the famous American radiobiologist J. Muller showed that ionizing radiation increased the rate of spontaneous mutations in animals. The problem is more complex for humans. The risk of genetic damage is very remote with doses lower than 1 or 2 Gy. No genetic effect was observed in the descendants of victims of Hiroshima and Nagasaki. (The embryonic malformations conferred to pregnant woman by ionizing radiation are obviously not in question here.) Furthermore, detection of genetic damage induced in astronauts by cosmic radiation is limited owing to the low number of subjects. It is worth pointing out that spontaneous mutations, which usually go undetected and are of no pathological consequence, affect more than 10% of the human population.

On the other hand, the fact that astronauts in space are obviously at higher risk explains the differences in the recommendations of the International Commission on Radiological Protection (ICRP). For terrestrial radiation workers, the annual dose limit is 50 mSv or 20 mSv, according to the new regulation. For astronauts, the maximum dose per year is 3 Sv. However, the difference is not so great if we consider the career dose limits: the dose for radiation workers is 2 Sv against 6 Sv for astronauts. Of course, the risk estimates and recommendations of the ICRP could be reviewed, taking into account various factors such as sex, age at exposure, or the level of neutrons inside the space station.

In spite of some uncertainties, it can be concluded that astronauts are exposed to a relatively low risk of radiation damage, at least during orbital flights. However, one has to have reservations on this issue due to problems related to solar flares, cosmic heavy ions and the possibility of a combined effect of microgravity and cosmic rays.

PROBLEMS RELATED TO COSMIC RADIATION

SOLAR FLARES

Solar flares are sudden, short-lived, light phenomena. Some are associated with large emissions of charged particles, in particular protons, and are called solar protonic events (SPE). SPEs last from 15 to 60 minutes. For humans, their most important feature is their variable intensity, which allows us to make a distinction between minor or ordinary and major or abnormally large protonic events.

Minor protonic events are frequent and occur several times a year. They are of low intensity and are responsible for a dose of only several tens or hundreds of mrad (the unit most often used to measure them). Minor events are of no danger. This is not the case, however, for major protonic events in which the sun abruptly emits an enormous flux of particles, on the order of $10^{10}/cm^2$ or more. The doses sent out into space vary from several tens to sometimes hundreds of rads. A solar event occurred in August 1972, resulting in a dose of approximately 500 rads (5 Gy) inside a spacecraft. We know that a dose of 450 rads or 4.5 Gy leads to death in 50% of irradiated individuals in 30 days. A very large protonic event could thus have catastrophic consequences during a manned space flight. Fortunately, such events are very rare since they occur approximately every four years. However, their danger is heightened by the fact that they are difficult to predict. They can be detected by early warning alarm systems only several minutes before the protonic flux hits. Major protonic events occur for the most part during periods of maximum solar activity, but the exact date of their occurrence and their amplitude cannot be predicted. These issues need to be further studied.

Solar protonic events normally pose no threat to human beings since the terrestrial atmosphere and the magnetosphere shield against them. The magnetosphere protects astronauts as well during low-orbit space missions. However, solar protonic events in particular abnormally large ones do constitute a serious risk for planetary, lunar and particularly Mars missions.

These missions will certainly be planned for periods when solar activity is at a minimum, but it is during theses periods that doses of galactic radiation are the highest. To limit this risk, astronauts should have access to a small, highly shielded area. This is possible though it will add extra weight to the spacecraft. Once on Mars or on the moon, astronauts could avoid the hazard of such major SPEs by constructing a shelter with planet soil. Exposure to cosmic radiation during round-trip missions over great distances obviously poses serious problems. Their importance should not be exaggerated, however, for it is likely that the psychological factor due to confinement, isolation and a certain level of stress will certainly play a more important role in the overall health of astronauts on long-term missions than cosmic radiation.

HEAVY COSMIC IONS

As mentioned earlier, heavy cosmic ions or HZE particles are atoms that have lost their electrons. These are the nuclei of atoms with an atomic number greater than 2. The most important are carbon, oxygen and iron. Their mass is much larger than that of other particles of cosmic radiation, and they remove more electrons from atoms and molecules than other types of radiation when they penetrate living matter. It is said that they have a great ionizing power. Their TEL[3] is often high, varying between a few keV/μ and 1000 keV/μ. The local doses are thus very high, often on the order of several grays or even several tens of grays.

Heavy ions can cause serious biological damage, leading eventually to cell death. Lethal damage is seen in cells that have been directly hit by one or several heavy particles (Figure 51). Sublethal lesions, to which cells survive, can also occur. These are caused by the electrons, which create an ionization cylinder several μm in

---

[3] In radiobiology, a radiation is characterized by the linear energy transferred per unit of track length (LET). The LET is usually expressed in keV/μm (kilo-electron volt/μm). A sparsely ionizing radiation, such as X-rays, has a low LET. The RBE increases rapidly with increasing LET but beyond a certain value the RBE falls, which corresponds to the overkill effect.

CONCEPT OF MICROLESION (GRAHN - TODD)

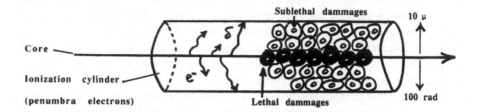

- A single particle can damage several cells.
- Biological effects can be detected for a single track.

FIGURE 51 *The microlesion concept*

A cell can be killed by a single heavy ion traveling through it. Many electrons, or δ rays, are ejected around the particle track and give rise to an ionizing cylinder called "penumbra." Cells irradiated by δ rays may survive, but the DNA damage can persist.
Doses inside the penumbra zone are much higher than the doses measured by global dosimetry.

diameter (thousandths of mm) around the trajectory of the particle. Many sublethal lesions to the DNA are poorly or not at all repaired. They persist during the entire lifetime of the cell and could be responsible for certain delayed responses. Such late effects will be discussed later. Despite its seriousness, the risk of biological damage is attenuated by the fact that heavy ions are comparatively rare, representing only 1% of all cosmic radiation particles. For instance, during the Biosatellite Cosmos flights, the number of heavy ions in the spacecraft was 6 per cm^2 per day. This very weak flux makes it difficult to determine their biological effects. Indeed, during a 2- to 3-week experiment, the proportion of cells of an organism directly hit by these particles is rather small. A technique to locate their path through an object has had to be developed in order to have a better understanding of their effects. One such technique used in my laboratory and in H. Bucker's laboratory in Germany consists in placing objects on a plate that is sandwiched between plastic sheets or nuclear emulsions acting as photographic film (Figure 52). The processing of the plastic foils and nuclear emulsions reveals the trajectories of heavy ions. The objects hit or missed can be studied separately. This technique was used for the first time during the Biostack 1 and 2 experiments aboard Apollo-16 and -17, using cysts from Artemia (Figure 53), a tiny shrimp found in many places throughout the planet as well as other biological material. The Artemia embryos inside the cysts can remain dormant for many years. When put back in seawater or an artificial medium, the cysts are rehydrated and their development is reactivated. The embryo hatches and is transformed into a tiny larva or nauplius that starts to swim in the culture medium.

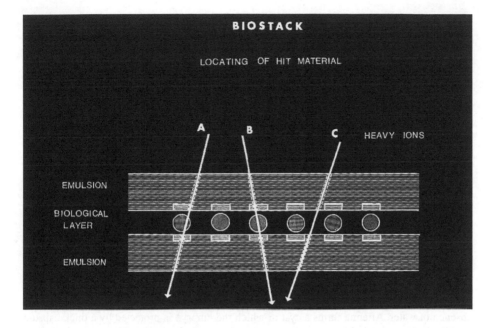

FIGURE 52 *The Biostack experiment*
In the American Biostack program and the Soviet Biorack program aboard their respective spacecrafts, the effects of cosmic heavy particles or heavy ions were investigated on small dormant organisms such as bacterial spores, eggs or seeds.
The biological organisms were embedded in polyvinylalcohol and the biological layer was sandwiched between detectors (plastic or nuclear emulsions). At the end of the experiment, the biological organisms, which had been hit or missed by heavy ions, were investigated.

The Biostack experiments demonstrated the severity of damage induced by heavy ions: a single particle can inhibit embryonic development (Figure 54). The same technique used in the BIOSTACK program or the BIOBLOC experiments aboard the Soviet Biocosmos satellites yielded additional results:

- Abnormal or completely arrested embryonic development in the *Carausius* insect
- Morphological abnormalities, such as the absence of roots in plantules grown from tobacco seeds (Figure 55)
- Chromosomal aberrations in lettuce embryos (studied at the Institute of Biomedical Problems in Moscow)
- Inactivation of *Bacillus subtilis* bacterial spores (studied by Gerda Horneck from the Institute of Aeronautic and Space Medicine in Cologne, Germany)

In these experiments it is clear that harmful effects were detected in objects hit by one or more heavy particles. However, developmental inhibition was also observed in the nonhit Artemia cysts though to a lesser extent than in cysts (*cf.* Figure 54) that

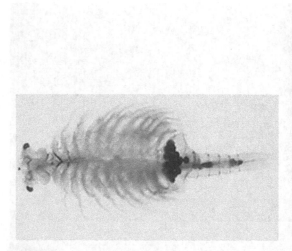
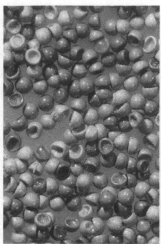

FIGRUE 53 *The Artemia shrimp (see Color figure X at the end of the book)*
This shrimp is present in seawater, particularly in California and in France (left); in the absence of water, Artemia forms a cyst in which the embryo is protected by a thick capsule (right); development is blocked and the embryo can remain dormant for many years. The embryos are reactivated when cysts are put back into seawater or in an artificial medium.

were hit. According to one hypothesis these responses were also linked to cosmic radiation but resulted from interactions between protons and living matter.

Many experiments performed on different subjects have demonstrated the harmful effects of heavy cosmic ions. But do humans experience similar effects? One piece of evidence to confirm this notion may be the light flashes that many astronauts have observed. During the Apollo flights, the astronauts claimed to have "seen" white or colored light flashes shaped like stars, lines or clouds when they were in the dark or when they had their eyes closed for several minutes. On Earth, these sensations can be caused by a small amount of pressure on the eyeball. Such light flashes have also been observed during other flights and occurred most often over the Southern Atlantic anomaly. These phenomena come from radiation. Indeed, their frequency is consistent with their being attributed to heavy ion fluxes. Furthermore, two courageous doctors from the Department of Biophysics at the University of California in Berkeley duplicated the appearance of this phenomenon using a heavy ion accelerator. They were indeed courageous because, although a retinal examination with an ophthalmoscope does not show lesions in astronauts, histological investigations using an electron microscope performed on rats after a three-week space flight have detected impressive tunnels dug inside the retina. It is likely that heavy ions were the source of this impressive damage (Figure 56).

The eye is not the only organ affected by heavy ions. Damage can appear in any organ and could be particularly serious for an organ such as the brain since most of its cells cannot be regenerated. Because of the great number of neurones in the central nervous system and the very weak flux of heavy ions, however, the risk is considered to be negligible for missions of several months or even several years.

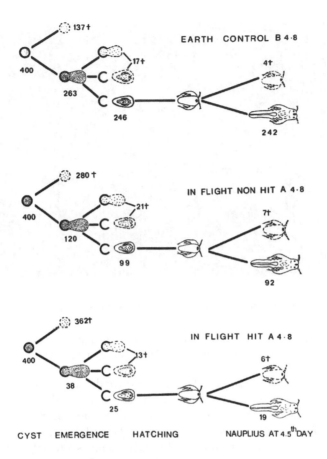

FIGRUE 54 *Results of the Biostack I experiment*

This experiment was carried out aboard Apollo-16 and repeated on the Apollo-17 mission (Dr. Bucker was the principal investigator). The figure illustrates the effects of space flight on Artemia cysts, which were hit or missed by a single heavy ion compared to the control.

In each case, the figure shows the number of cysts hatching and those developing into viable nauplii (larvae) on the fourth day of the experiment. The results demonstrate the lethal effects of a single heavy ion on an Artemia cyst.

THE COMBINED EFFECT OF COSMIC RADIATION AND WEIGHTLESSNESS

DNA repair is an essential cellular function. Indeed, even in the absence of radiation, normal cell metabolism continually alters DNA structure, making repairs that are crucial to cell survival. It is possible that this function is disturbed in a weightless environment. If this were the case, then radioprotection recommendations based on ground-based research would not be adequate for astronautics.

Several experiments investigating DNA repair under microgravity have been carried out in the past. Organisms were irradiated using an identical radioactive source with doses much higher than those given out by cosmic rays. The flight subjects showed more damage than ground control subjects. These results suggest

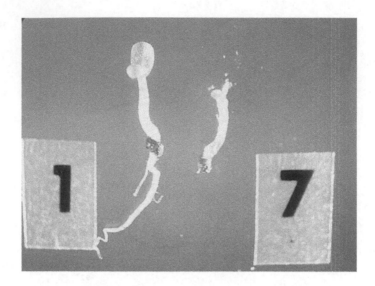

FIGURE 55 *Biological effects of cosmic heavy ions (see Color figure XI at the end of the book)*

Irradiation of a tobacco seed by a single heavy ion can induce abnormalities in the development of the seedling. The figure shows an absence of root. (Pr. Delpoux, University of Toulouse.)

that the space flight increased the effects of cosmic radiation. This phenomenon has been observed in seeds as well as Drosophila. In addition, the effects of artificial bone marrow irradiation were more pronounced for rats aboard the Soviet Cosmos-690 satellite than for control groups irradiated on the ground. However, not all research points to these conclusions. German and Czech scientists studied *Escherichia coli* bacteria and human fibroblast cells on the Spacelab IML-2 mission. They irradiated cells with high doses of X- and gamma rays before the flight. The study of radiation-induced DNA damage and cell survival showed that irradiation affected both cell types similarly. It can be concluded that the DNA repair mechanisms were not modified by microgravity (Horneck, G., 1999). This potentially important finding should be explored in future research.

Delayed or Late Effects

In addition to immediate biological damage, ionizing radiation can cause damage that only appears years after irradiation. Such late effects often involve a decrease in life span. Early radiologists, who were unaware of the hazards of radiation or the basic rules of radioprotection, suffered the consequences. Investigations were also carried out in Drosophila. A space flight of several weeks resulted in a decrease in their life span but weightlessness seems to have been the primary cause in this case. Since astronautics is a recently developed field, possible effects on life span in man are still unknown.

Genetic and carcinogenic effects are also late effects of radiation. As was previously reported, the risk of genetic and carcinogenic effects seems to be very low

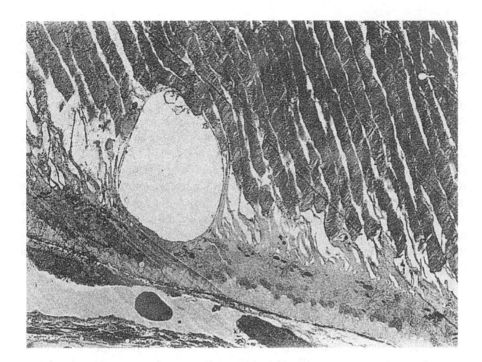

FIGURE 56 *Biological effects of cosmic heavy ions*
The electron micrograph of a rat retina after a space flight shows holes probably produced by cosmic heavy ions. Damage was also noted in accelerator experiments after irradiation with heavy ions (D. Philpott *et al.*).

in astronauts. However, the suggestion that the risk caused by cosmic rays is minimal was based on total radiation doses, which are always low. As we have come to understand heavy ions and the importance of their energy losses to living matter in greater depth, it has become clear that there is a large discrepancy between radiation doses measured by global dosimetry and those measured locally (microdosimetry). Local doses along the tracks of the HZE particles are much higher. In light of this fact, it would be wise to reconsider the possible genetic and cancer risks of cosmic radiation.

Experimental evidence raises questions about genetic effects induced by cosmic radiation. Genetic effects have often been reported in plants and animals after space flights. Studies, including the one performed by R. Hara from the University of Kyoto on the IML-2 Shuttle mission, have shown an increase in the incidence of mutations in *Bacillus subtilis* and Drosophila. In addition, mutations have been observed in tobacco plantules and in *Arabidopsis*, a plant often used in space biology. The fact that much higher doses of X or gamma radiation are required to induce comparable genetic effects on Earth suggests that cosmic heavy ions could be responsible for such effects. In space, the most pronounced mutational effects have indeed been detected in subjects hit by one or more heavy particles or in those situated near their tracks.

This evidence calls for an examination of the possibility that heavy cosmic ions might cause genetic damage in humans. However, calculations based on missions lasting a couple of months show that the risk of genetic effect in the descendants of astronauts is negligible. For this to occur, one of the immature sex cells in the testes or ovaries would need to be damaged by a heavy ion impact. The probability of this occurring is very low. Since the effect of missions lasting several years or repeated missions are unknown, a cautious attitude is therefore warranted.

Heavy ions might also increase the incidence of cancer and leukemia. We know that electrons ejected along the tracks of heavy ions can cause sublethal damage to DNA. If this damage persists, it could in time cause the injured cells to be transformed into neoplastic cells. (Transformed cells proliferate rapidly and can cause tumors when injected into susceptible animal hosts.) This notion is supported by experimental evidence: on Earth, heavy ion irradiation can lead to the transformation of cells cultivated *in vitro*. High-energy ions, which are similar to cosmic heavy ions, cause the most damage. Furthermore, their carcinogenic effect is greater for low-rate than for high-rate irradiation at the same dose, and astronauts are exposed to continuous radiation at very low dose rate.

In summary, it is not yet known what effect heavy particle radiation will have on humans during space flight missions lasting several months or even years, but the irradiation damage seen *in vitro* is disturbing. Although the incidence of cancer in astronauts has remained unchanged up to this point, the risks they are exposed to due to cosmic radiation will not be fully characterized for several years. Nevertheless, the risk is probably only associated with very long-term missions.

CONCLUSION

In summary, men in space are exposed to natural radiation from cosmic rays at doses that are much higher than those found on Earth. However, risks on current missions are limited, especially in the case of ISS missions. For long-term missions, on the other hand, all the problems are clearly not resolved. Studies are in progress and additional investigations must be carried out in the future to ensure that cosmic rays do not become a limiting factor, especially for very long missions.

14 Extraterrestrial Life

Until recently exobiology referred to the study of life in places other than Earth itself. Today, the terms of astrobiology and bioastronomy refer to the same field. These disciplines are close to space biology, the purpose of which goes beyond the mere observation and analysis of organisms launched into space. Space biology also aims to explore the possibility of extraterrestrial life. It is conceivable that other organisms could have developed in surroundings completely different from ours.

Anticipating that such organisms will one day be discovered, astrobiological research focuses on creatures that are considered alive due to their ability to acclimatize, reproduce, synthesize and self-regulate, regardless of form, size or ability to react to signals from the external world. Extraterrestrial beings might be similar to Earth-based life forms, that is, made out of proteins (themselves made of amino acids), fats (lipids), sugars and starches, mineral elements and water, which represents two thirds of human body weight. Three molecules play a fundamental role in living matter: DNA (deoxyribonucleic acid), the subsections of which are individual genes; RNA (ribonucleic acid), which is responsible for protein synthesis; and ATP (adenosine triphosphate) the degradation of which releases the energy necessary for cellular metabolism, movement and reproduction.

The majority of these carbon-based organic compounds can be synthesized *in vitro* by successively adding molecules made up of atoms of hydrogen, carbon, nitrogen and oxygen to form large molecules. It is likely that these molecules were the precursors of life on Earth some 3.8 to 3.5 billion years ago, hence the name prebiotic compounds.

Thus astrobiology not only seeks extant forms of extraterrestrial life, but also looks for the possibility that life may develop. Prebiotic compounds represent the chance that living organisms have existed or will exist on other planets.

LIFE IN THE SOLAR SYSTEM

It makes sense to search for extraterrestrial life within our solar system first even if the chances of finding it are slim. Theoretically, the greatest probability of success is with Mars or Titan.

MARS

The existence of Mars has been recognized since antiquity and the Greeks associated the planet with the God of war. Later, Mars, like the other planets, was believed to be inhabited. This idea was reinforced in the late 19th century when Percival Lowell and Giovanni Virginio Schiaparelli in 1882 claimed to have seen numerous straight lines they interpreted as irrigation canals running across Mars continents from one sea to another. In their opinion, such formations could only be the work of intelligent beings. Of course, the two astronomers were using low-resolution telescopes. All the same, these ideas persisted for many years until space probes were able to explore the surface of the red planet.

Since the beginning of astronautics, Mars has been the focus of exploration. The limited data available about this planet could be construed as evidence that it contained traces of life. After the launch of a Soviet probe in 1952, the American Mariner probes used between 1965 and 1971 showed that the entire surface was rocky and devoid of water. The atmosphere of Mars is very thin and very different from the atmosphere of our planet. It is comprised of 96% carbon dioxide, whereas the terrestrial atmosphere contains 78% nitrogen, a little argon and 21% oxygen. Could more simple life forms such as microorganisms live buried in the soil of Mars, thus partially protected from the very low temperatures prevailing on the red planet? The American biologist Albert Taylor jokingly suggested using a mousetrap and a camera as a means of exploring the planet. Harold Klein and his colleagues took a more rational approach. They recommended using a highly sensitive technique to look for organic compounds and evidence of metabolic processes, particularly in the form of gaseous exchanges, which would indicate the presence of living beings. The Viking mission was designed with these two objectives in mind.

Two missions, each comprising a craft to orbit Mars (Orbiter) and a probe to land on the Martian surface (Lander) took place at a 2.5-month interval in 1976. Upon reaching Mars, the Landers separated from the Orbiters at an altitude of 1,500 km. At 6,000 m, they deployed their parachutes, which were then detached at 1,500 m above the Martian surface. The use of retrorockets allowed for a soft landing.

The first probe, Viking Lander-1, landed on July 20, 1976 on the Chryse Planitia in the Martian northern hemisphere. The second probe, Viking Lander-2, landed on September 3 on the Utopia Planitia, on the opposite side of the planet, 1,500 km further north. Each probe weighed 390 kg and was equipped with two cameras, extremely sophisticated instruments and a mechanical arm for soil sample collection.

Three experiments were designed to detect evidence of life, especially micro-organisms. The experiments were each performed several times since the Viking probes were able to function for a number of months. In fact, Viking-1 continued to function for 6 years, even though the scientific program had only been designed to last 90 days. The purpose of the Viking experimental mission was to detect metabolic activity, i.e., absorption capacity, synthesis and excretion (Figure 57).

The first experiment, named PR for pyrolysis release, tested for bacterial life in the Martian soil. If bacteria capable of photosynthesis were exposed to carbon dioxide and light, they should synthesize organic compounds. On Earth, some bacteria, algae and most plants perform this type of reaction daily. They use solar energy to synthesize numerous organic substances from atmospheric carbon dioxide.

Martian soil samples were exposed to carbon monoxide and carbon dioxide, both of which were labeled with radioactive carbon (^{14}C). A xenon lamp simulated solar light. After 120 hours, the radioactive gases were expelled, the lamp turned off and the sample heated to a temperature of 625°C to perform a pyrolysis. The latter breaks

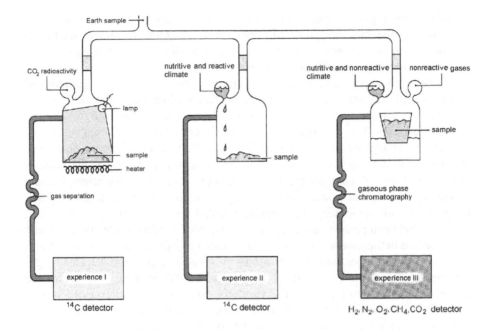

FIGURE 57 *Experiments from the Viking missions (see Color figure XII at the end of the book)*

In experiment 1 (pyrolyse release or PR), a sample of Martian soil was exposed to radioactive CO_2 and light. In experiment 2 (labeled release or LR) the sample was put in contact with a radioactive labeled culture medium generally used to grow bacteria in the laboratory. In experiment 3 (gaseous exchange or GEx), the composition of the atmosphere in the container was studied after adding water vapor or nutrient medium.

down organic matter into water and carbon dioxide. Any released radioactive gas would have to come from ^{14}C-labeled organic matter, thus providing evidence that Martian soil contained bacteria. Viking-1 performed this experiment soon after landing and did find that radioactive carbon dioxide had been released. Scientists thus claimed that they had found Martian microorganisms capable of photosynthesis.

The second experiment, named LR for labeled release, was similar to the first except that in this case a nutrient medium containing the ^{14}C-labeled organic acids, formic and lactic acids, as well as amino acids such as glycine and alanine, were added to the chamber. (A similar medium is used to cultivate bacteria in the laboratory.) These substances had been chosen because they appear to have been formed before life began on Earth and because they might be available on Mars as building blocks for living organisms.

A Martian soil sample was exposed to this medium at 10°C. If the sample contained microorganisms, the latter would absorb this nutritive soup and metabolically convert part of it to carbon dioxide, which they could then expel. Since the initial nutrients were radioactive, the carbon dioxide would also be labeled. Here again, the experiment seemed to be successful. The gaseous atmosphere became richer in radioactive carbon. It thus appeared that the bacteria had released carbon dioxide, a seemingly indisputable proof of metabolic activity. This was apparently confirmed by the fact that preheating the sample to 145°C for 3.5 hours before testing the sample suppressed the release of carbon dioxide. At that temperature, any microorganisms would have been destroyed.

In the third experiment, named GEx for gaseous exchange, the Martian soil sample was placed in a small hermetically closed container filled with water vapor. This was an attempt to simulate an environment that might have existed two or three billion years ago. The first phase of the experiment caused an abrupt release of oxygen, increasing the oxygen present 200-fold. Terrestrial organisms capable of photosynthetic activity do release oxygen, but in a slow and progressive fashion. The second phase of the experiment was carried out after adding a nutrient medium rich in amino acids and vitamins as well as a gaseous atmosphere containing helium, krypton and carbon dioxide. The experiment lasted seven months.

If life had been present, this long incubation period would have led to significant modifications in the gaseous atmosphere since metabolically active organisms absorb and release gaseous compounds. Unfortunately, no change could be detected by gas chromatography at the end of the incubation period. Given these new results, the first experiments were repeated. The pyrolysis experiment was performed several times, but the results of the experiment could never be duplicated. The second experiment had made one believe that Martian bacteria could use a nutrient medium. Thus adding this medium again should have caused the bacteria to release more carbon dioxide. But this second attempt was negative.

The Viking probes were equipped with extremely sensitive mass spectrometers coupled to gas chromatographs to identify the molecules in a gaseous mixture. They could detect organic molecules containing more than two carbon atoms, even though their mass might be only a billionth of the total mass of the sample under investigation. Despite this remarkable capacity, the Viking spectrometer only detected minute quantities of organic substances originating from the solvents used for cleaning the machine when it had been built. It is clear that the sensitivity threshold of these instruments was too high to detect compounds originating directly from living bacteria. But why would they not be capable of detecting organic products accumulated by successive generations of bacteria. The only explanation for the negative results is that an exceptional phenomenon exists on the surface of Mars that causes the degradation of all organic compounds. This hypothesis remains to be proven, however.

If living organisms were not present on Mars, how could the seemingly positive results of the first experiments be explained? The answer is simple: the results were due to iron oxides and peroxides, which are found in abundance on the surface of rocks scattered about Mars. These compounds are extremely reactive and give out oxygen in the presence of water, as had occurred in the GEx experiment. They fixed the carbon monoxide in the PR experiment, thus explaining the detection of a radioactive gas. Moreover, the GEx and LR experiments gave the same results when repeated on Earth using peroxides in the absence of living organisms.

The Viking experiments demonstrated chemosynthesis phenomena rather than biosynthesis. However, these experiments do not eliminate the possibility that living beings or fossil forms exist on Mars. Photographs taken by Mariner-9 and the Viking mission craft that orbited Mars led to a remarkable discovery. A series of sinuous

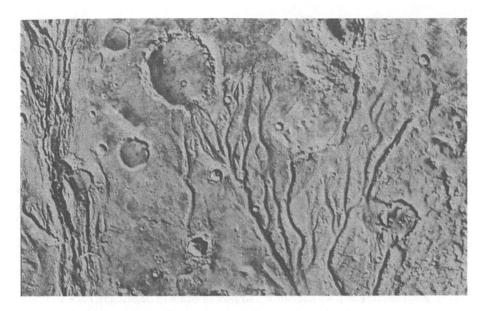

FIGURE 58 *The surface of Mars*
The surface of Mars is dry, but the pictures taken during the Viking missions and, later, by Mars Observer suggest there once was an ancient river network. At the moment, ice is present in the polar regions of Mars and deep below the planet's surface.

valleys, a kilometer wide and several hundreds of kilometers long, can be seen on the surface of the planet. Their pattern points to the existence of an ancient river network that dried up long ago (Figure 58). The occasional recurrence of water might have resulted from short periods of atmospheric warming, giving rise to seas and oceans. The nature of rocks on Mars also supports the theory that water was once present on the planet. These rocks contain clay-like minerals and salts similar to those found on Earth and formed only in the presence of water. Their formation would have occurred sometime between the early ages of the planet and 3.5 billion years ago. A white cap at the Martian North Pole is composed of frozen water (and CO_2 probably), as is the permafrost, the layer of frozen soil deep below the planet's surface.

The above evidence reinforces the possibility that life may have once existed on Mars. It is feasible that, given the presence of liquid water, life might have appeared on Mars during the same era that it did on Earth. When the planet later cooled down, all life would have disappeared. Traces of organic compounds or fossils might still be discovered deep in the sedimentary layers of lakes and ancient seas. One might even discover organisms in the cyst form safely buried in the Martian subsoil when the planet cooled down. Such organisms could perhaps be revived upon contact with a warm and humid atmosphere.

While the debate continues, further missions to Mars have been carried out. On July 4, 1997, the Mars Pathfinder probe landed on the red planet. This successful mission followed two failed missions, that of Mars Observer, which disappeared in August 1993, and that of the Mars-96 probe, which was damaged over the Pacific Ocean in November 1996 without ever having left Earth's orbit.

The success of Mars Pathfinder was remarkable. After landing, the probe released Sojourner, a robot weighing only 11.5 kg. Sojourner traveled at a speed of 40 cm per minute and was equipped with a camera, a small lithium battery, and an X-ray and proton spectrometer built by scientists at the Max Planck Institute in Mainz and the University of Chicago. The Martian surface temperature was milder during this mission than during the Viking missions: on the order of –12°C rather than –75°C. Sojourner's task included bombarding Martian rocks with alpha particles and analyzing their chemical composition based on the reflected spectra. Pathfinder landed at the bottom of a large valley, the Ares Vallis, where the soil was strewn with rocks facing the same direction and separated by what seemed to be small grains of sand. It was as if water had run through the valley 3 to 3.5 billion years before, a hypothesis consistent with the analysis performed by Sojourner's spectrometer: the rocks contained quartz, a mineral formed in the presence of water. The photographs taken recently by Mars Global Surveyor show what appears to be traces of streams going back a million years ago, according to some, and possibly less than ten thousand years according to Kenneth Edgett.

Amongst the missions planned for the beginning of this century, Mars Surveyor-5 is of great interest as it should allow samples of Mars to be brought back to Earth for study. Unfortunately, the recovery of such samples has been recently postponed to 2014, 2015 or even later.

In addition to the research on Mars, other studies have been carried out on Earth in an attempt to determine whether extreme climate conditions, such as those on Mars, are compatible with life. Expeditions to Antarctica by numerous scientists, including Christopher McKey, have shown that life could exist in regions as inhospitable as Mars. Lichens, a symbiotic association of algae, fungi and photosynthetic bacteria, have been discovered in the rocky rims of Antarctic valleys. Algae have been found at the bottom of frozen lakes, living at temperatures as low as –20°C. This type of finding shows that life can indeed exist in such harsh environment, and Mars could be one such environment.

Other research conducted on the ground involves meteorites originating from Mars. These controversial studies will be discussed later.

TITAN: A MODEL OF PREBIOTIC SYNTHESIS ON EARTH?

Titan is one of Saturn's moons. Owing to its considerable size, Christiaan Huygens was able to discover it as early as 1655. The equatorial diameter of Titan is 4,900 km, while that of Saturn is roughly 121,000 km and that of Earth about 12,760 km. Titan is the only celestial body in the solar system with an atmosphere rich in nitrogen and an atmospheric pressure similar to Earth's (1.5 bar).

When the Voyager-1 probe flew by Titan at a distance of less than 7,000 km in November 1980, it found that its atmosphere also contained methane, probably argon, and various hydrocarbons such as methyl acetylene, formed from the action of UV solar radiation on methane. Most importantly, Voyager-1 and its infrared spectrometer revealed the presence of atmospheric nitrogen compounds such as hydrocyanic acid. This compound is of major importance amongst prebiotic compounds as it could be the starting point for the synthesis of amino acids (Figure 59).

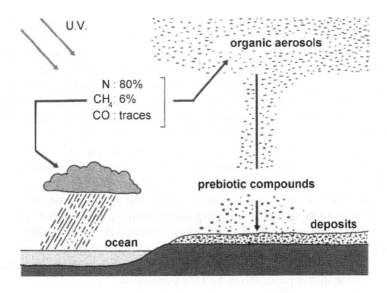

FIGURE 59 *Diagram showing the atmosphere and surface of Titan*

Titan, a moon of Saturn, is of great interest to astrobiologists. Its atmosphere contains methane and various hydrocarbons. Methane (or ethane) can precipitate in the form of rain and thus give rise to oceans. Prebiotic organic compounds originating from aerosols in the atmosphere continuously precipitate and form a thick sediment layer on the surface of Titan. The extreme cold on Titan has preserved these organic compounds, like food in a freezer. (From Planel, H. *L'Espace et la Vie*. Larousse, Paris, 1988.)

It is possible that the methane on Titan precipitated on the ground in the form of rain, thus giving rise to methane and ethane oceans. Furthermore, the organic products might form a thick cloudy layer, aerosol-like in structure, situated at an altitude of approximately 300 km. The molecules, isolated or agglomerated, would constantly fall and thus form a kind of sedimentary layer several hundred meters thick.

Despite the presence of organic molecules on Titan, it is unlikely that life exists on this moon. For one thing it contains no water, a crucial factor in the appearance of life as it is known on Earth. The other reason is the very low surface temperature of −180°C.

In spite of this, there is considerable interest in Titan. A mission to this moon might reveal organic compounds that, given more favorable conditions, would combine to form living matter on Earth. The extreme cold on Titan has prevented such evolution but might, on the other hand, have conserved prebiotic compounds like a giant freezer.

To explore these theories further, scientists launched the Huygens Cassini mission in October 1997. The mission, due to last almost seven years, consists of a probe aimed directly at Titan. It was named after the Dutchman Christiaan Huygens who discovered Titan and the Italian astronomer, Jean-Dominique Cassini who discovered four of Saturn's other satellites and the gaps between its rings. Huygens and Cassini, both attracted by the glory of the sun King Louis XIV, came to settle in Paris. Indeed, the Cassini family directed the Paris Observatory for four generations.

The Huygens Cassini mission consists of two parts: the Cassini spacecraft, constructed by NASA, and the Huygens probe, built by the European Space Agency. During its nearly seven-year voyage, the spacecraft is programmed to fly by the Earth, Venus and Jupiter, and use the gravitational fields of these planets to propel itself toward Saturn. Upon entering Saturn's orbit in July 2004, the Cassini spacecraft will release the Huygens probe. As the probe approaches the surface of Titan, the moon's dense atmosphere, which is five times that of the Earth, will heat the probe shield to a temperature of approximately 1800°C. Once on the surface, the probe should be able to resist the very low temperatures for several minutes. During this time, a mass spectrometer and gas chromatograph will study Titan's atmosphere and provide data about the chemical composition of the soil and the presence of methane. Photographs will be taken and the temperature will be measured to 0.1°C. An acoustical detector on the probe will help determine the nature of Titan's surface: a "bang" indicating a hard surface and a "plop" meaning the probe landed on a sea. The data will be transmitted back to Earth by the orbiting Cassini spacecraft, which will also photograph and study Saturn, its rings and its 17 other moons. Nevertheless, Titan is the one that is most intriguing for exobiologists.

BEYOND MARS AND TITAN

Titan is not the only celestial body in the solar system to contain prebiotic compounds or organic molecules. There are such compounds on Jupiter and Saturn. Although the conditions that prevail on Jupiter hardly seem conducive to the development of living matter, the American astronomer Carl Sagan imagined the existence of extraordinary Jovian beings that resemble hot-air balloons and move about the planet's atmosphere using organic compounds formed at their level. Indeed, Jupiter has a dense, rocky and extremely hot core surrounded by a thick gaseous cloud made up of 90% hydrogen and 10% helium. Its atmosphere is made up of methane, ethylene, acetylene, nitrogen, ammonia and even traces of water vapor that have been detected in the upper layers. Prebiotic synthesis might have given birth to strange life forms moving about the atmosphere in areas where the temperature hovers around 0°C, which is definitely milder than the −150°C that prevail on the planet's "surface." Should Sagan be followed in his flights of fancy? In reality, the probability of life is extremely remote, since the Jovian atmosphere is home to constant currents that probably push all the organic compounds formed within it toward the lower layers where the temperature must break them down into simpler compounds.

Even though Venus is a much better explored planet, it is also a poor candidate for extraterrestrial life. Venus has been visited several times by the American Pioneer and Soviet Venera probes. The results of these missions in conjunction with the data already collected from Earth-based observations were very disappointing. The atmosphere surrounding Venus consists of 75 to 80% sulphuric acid droplets. Moreover, its surface cannot contain water because the temperature, which is about 450°C, is too high. This is due to a greenhouse effect. Indeed, below the sulphuric acid cloud, the gaseous atmosphere essentially made up of carbon dioxide retains the heat given off at the surface of Venus.

Despite such inhospitable conditions, there is still the chance that life developed in the solar system elsewhere than on Earth. There are bacteria able to adapt to remarkably hostile environments such as the polar regions. The bacterium *Micrococcus radiodurans* has been isolated in the coolant water of a nuclear reactor. Its lethal dose (LD 50) is on the order of 1 million rads! Others have been discovered in extraordinary places such as concentrated solutions of sulphuric acid or solid plastics. Extreme temperatures do not seem to be an obstacle for certain life forms: marine archeobacteria were recently discovered at a depth of 2,600 m above underwater volcanoes near the East Pacific Rise. They have also been found in the sulphur-rich hot springs along the island of Vulcano off the coast of Sicily. These anaerobic bacteria survive deep in the sea despite temperatures ranging between 110 and 120°C and pressures of up to 250 atmospheres. Such bacteria are probably comparable to the primitive species that appeared on the Earth more than 3 billion years ago. At that time, active volcanoes covered the Earth's surface, and the atmosphere was practically devoid of oxygen. Similar species might exist on other planets, on a moon such as Io, where the Voyager probe discovered volcanic activity in the spring of 1979.

Finally, the Jupiter satellite, Europe, could contain life forms present in liquid water under the thick layer of ice detected on photographs taken by the Galileo probe.

METEORITES AND COMETS

The solar system does not only contain planets and their moons, but meteorites, asteroids and comets as well. Although they do not contain living matter, they are still of interest to biologists.

The Earth is constantly showered with meteorites that break apart in the upper atmosphere. On February 12, 1947, a disintegrating meteorite created 120 craters, 375 km from Vladivostock. Other larger meteorite craters exist, such as the one discovered in Arizona by pioneers in the 1870s; the over 1 km-wide crater was dug by a meteorite that fell some 50,000 years ago. Fortunately, Siberia and Arizona were uninhabited at the time. The Hoba meteorite that fell in South Africa in 1920 weighed 60 tons. In the past, meteorites that were several kilometers in diameter led to the disappearance of most living creatures, 251 and 65.5 million year ago.

A good number of meteorites originate from asteroids in the asteroid belt between the orbits of Jupiter and Mars. Asteroids orbit the sun and were probably formed at the same time as the rest of the solar system. Meteorites are fragments that break off an asteroid after a collision. The fragments can be more than 200 km in diameter.

Some of the meteorites that have fallen on Earth, such as the one that landed on the French village of Orgueil in 1864, have been thought to contain extraterrestrial life forms. In fact, this meteorite was contaminated with bacteria and yeast from the terrestrial soil. More recently, better-preserved meteorites were found in Antarctica. These rocks are composed of carbonized chondrites but, interestingly, contain compounds such as amino acids as well as purine and pyrimidine bases. These bases are found in the nucleic acids that make up DNA. It is very unlikely that the prebiotic molecules found on these meteorites are due to contamination since they are slightly different from the organic compounds found in terrestrial living matter. When amino acids from Earth-based life forms are put in solution and illuminated with polarized light, the light is deviated to the left; they are said to be of the "L" form. Among the amino acids found on the meteorite, half behaved in a similar manner, while the other half caused the light to deviate to the right and are therefore the "D" form of the molecule. Thus it is likely that the amino acids found in these meteorites did not originate from terrestrial contamination, and that prebiotic synthesis occurred in another part of the solar system some 4 billion years ago.

Meteorites could provide further evidence for the existence of extraterrestrial life in the solar system. Several meteorites that originated from the planet Mars are available for study. One of these, ALH84001, weighs nearly 2 kg and was discovered by Allan Hills in the ice of the Antarctic in 1995. The impact of a large meteorite probably broke this piece of rock off the bottom of a Martian crater some 1.6 billion years ago. The crater, itself 3.6 billion years old, might have been filled with water and could have been a likely site for the development of primitive life. After the water disappeared, fossils might have remained. It is a rather impressive scenario, according to David MacKay, especially if the vestiges of primitive life are discovered on the meteorite. They would include compounds belonging to the PAH family, a group of complex aromatic hydrocarbons which might have biological origins as well as carbonate compound globules. On the other hand, scanning electron microscope images of the rock have led to the spectacular discovery of elongated forms that MacKay believes to be bacterial fossils or nanobacteria (Figure 60).

Unfortunately, this evidence is not definitive proof of extra terrestrial life. The interpretation which MacKay and his team published were met with severe criticism. Some astrobiologists pointed out that the forms taken to be fossilized bacteria are much smaller in size (0.1 μm) than the terrestrial bacteria found today. In addition, the structure of the PAH found in the meteorite seems too simple to be of biological origin. Finally, it is possible that this meteorite, which supposedly traveled 16 million years and remained buried in Antarctic ice for more than 10,000 years, was contaminated. Similar forms of PAH have been discovered in the ice where Alan Hills found the meteorite.

It is also possible that the microscopic rod-shaped structures found in the meteorite are of terrestrial origin. Indeed, in the early 1990s, a Finish biologist discovered nanobacteria in the ground that were 20 or a 100 times smaller than already known bacteria. Later on, nanobacteria were even found in human blood and in gallbladder stones. Both these discoveries lead one to question the data on the Martian meteorite bacterial fossils. Furthermore, scientists have observed such structures in the fragments of a meteorite that fell in Tunisia near Tatahouine in 1931 and that were collected for study 63 years later. However, no such structures were observed in fragments studied as soon as they hit the Earth. The same is true of fragments conserved in laboratories. Despite the public excitement concerning ALH84001 and the possibility of extraterrestrial life, such data should be interpreted with caution.

Comets are among the most beautiful celestial bodies in the sky. They were formed, like asteroids, at the same time as the rest of the solar system and are concentrated in the Oort cloud at the far reaches of the solar system. Comets occasionally exit the Oort cloud and leave the solar system or move toward the sun. They become visible

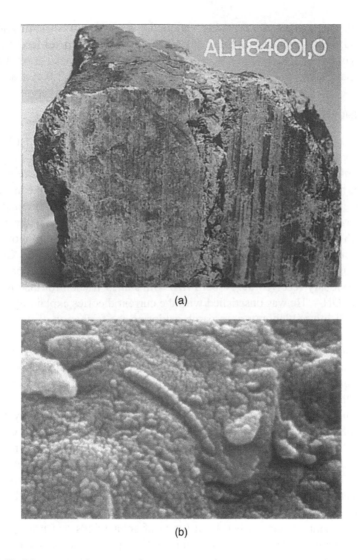

(a)

(b)

FIGURE 60 *Mars meteorite*

a) The meteorite ALH 84001, weighing nearly 2 kg and discovered in the ice of the Antarctic in 1995, is probably of Martian origin (NASA).

b) Investigations carried out by David MacKay support the idea that there are primitive life forms. Scanning microscope studies have led to the discovery of elongated forms considered to be fossils of nanobacteria. Such nanobacteria, 20 to 100 times smaller than most bacteria, have been recently discovered on Earth.

to us as they approach the Earth. A comet has a nucleus only several kilometers long composed of ice covered by carbonated granules. When a comet approaches the sun part of its ice vaporizes or sublimates. The comet is then surrounded by a kind of cloud or tail made of dust and hydroxyl ions (OH). The latter originate from the decomposition of water (H_2O) under the action of UV radiation. The tail and probably the nucleus contain organic compounds such as methyl cyanide and hydro-cyanic acid. In spite of the fact that these compounds are very different from the molecules of living matter, comet nuclei are more than mere blocks of ice. Chemical reactions have taken place there as they have in other regions of the solar system.

Life Outside the Solar System

Let us now think beyond the solar system and discuss the possibility that life, either primitive or evolved, exists elsewhere in the universe. Some theories propose that life on Earth originated in space. This is known as panspermia. It is an old theory that comes back into fashion periodically but remains in the realm of the unverifiable. Curiously enough, some of its strongest proponents are renowned scientists.

The Swedish chemist S.A. Arrhenius put forward this hypothesis at the beginning of the 20th century. He was awarded the Nobel Prize for research showing how molecules in solution dissociate into ions. Several decades later, Francis Crick gave new impetus to the theory of panspermia with the concept of managed panspermia. He had previously received the Nobel Prize with James Watson for discovering the structure of DNA. He was unsatisfied with the current theories explaining the origin of life and dismissed laboratory research exploring the formation of proto-DNA or RNA from organic compounds. The latter experiments suggest that the precursors of biological molecules could have formed in oceans, lakes or lagoons. Crick instead believed that the Earth had been seeded with several billion bacteria brought by a spaceship originating from a faraway planet inhabited by a highly evolved civiliza-tion. This ship would have drifted for 10,000 years or more propelled by solar wind pressure on a large, extremely thin sail. The latter concept is actually based on reality: indeed, a solar sail project has actually been discussed in some countries.

Along the same lines, other theories suggest that bacterial spores might have traveled millions of years through space and reached the Earth, albeit not in a spaceship. Terrestrial spores are in a cyst form that is particularly resistant. It is possible that spores on some distant planet might have been ejected from their natural habitat by a comet or meteorite impact. Once propelled into space, they might have traveled from star to star, pushed by a series of solar winds and protected by the clouds of organic molecules found in interstellar space. Laboratory experiments effectively demonstrate that bacterial spores can resist a vacuum, UV radiation and a temperature close to $-263°C$ for long periods of time. However, spores might not be able to withstand the elevated doses of cosmic radiation in space. The panspermia hypothesis therefore remains a grand hypothesis.

In recent years, public belief in extraterrestrial life has increased significantly. The belief in extraterrestrial UFOs (unidentified flying objects) visiting Earth is also more common. This phenomenon has been exhaustively debated and even NASA has been involved to some extent in its exploration. Astronauts claimed to have observed UFOs, particularly in the early years of manned space flights. MacDivitt supposedly observed and photographed UFOs during the Gemini-4 flight in June 1965. However, what he saw was nothing more than the last stage of the booster rocket. The luminous object that Charles Conrad photographed aboard Gemini-2 was in fact the Soviet Proton satellite-3 just before it disappeared into the terrestrial atmosphere. Similarly, Apollo astronauts claimed to have seen UFOs during the lunar missions. Here, again, these sightings proved to be nothing more than fragments of the Saturn rocket that had launched the space vehicle. None of these claims have stood up to close scrutiny.

In addition to sightings in space, numerous UFOs have supposedly been observed on the ground. However, none of the evidence concerning these encounters is compelling enough to verify whether UFOs do indeed exist. With as many cameras in the United States as there are citizens, only a stroke of incredibly bad luck could explain the lack of an irrefutable piece of evidence. One document considered proof that extraterrestrial beings do exist seems in fact to be a photograph of a burned monkey, a passenger aboard a U.S. army rocket that crashed in Mexico on July 7, 1948. As for the phenomena observed in Rockwell, the poor image quality and the otherwise unthinkable silence of the government and scientific authorities can only lead one to argue against the existence of UFOs.

As for extraterrestrial ships disappearing suddenly into the sky and moving faster than the speed of light... it is difficult to believe in something that so completely denies the laws of physics. Finally, it is improbable that visitors in all likelihood endowed with extraordinary means of communication would pass right by us without leaving a message. We, on the other hand, have made efforts to attempt such communication: the American Pioneer-10 and -11 probes carry a plaque engraved with a message destined to inform possible inhabitants of other planets about our civilization on Earth (Figure 61). Likewise, the Voyager probes each have a disk

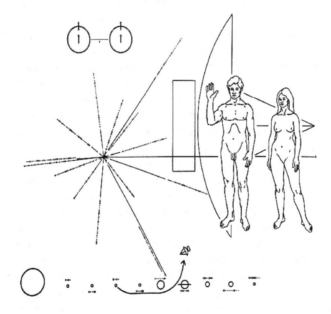

FIGURE 61 *The Pioneer message*

Launched in 1972, Pioneer-10 was the first probe to leave the solar system. Pioneer-10 carried a message engraved on a small aluminum plate. This message contains (from left to right and from top to bottom): the hydrogen atom, pulsars directed from the Sun, the planets of the solar system and drawings of the spatial probe, a man and a woman.

carrying information, cordial messages and greetings from the President of the United States. Anyone able to decipher it will know without a doubt that they are not alone in the universe.

Molecules in Space

A more scientific examination of whether extraterrestrial life exists might lead to a greater understanding of life in space. Given current technological means, can we detect life in the universe or in our galaxy? This is an enormous task according to astronomer Jean Heidemann since our galaxy spans 100,000 billion times the distance between New York and Paris. There are nearly 200 billion stars in our galaxy, some of them possibly harboring an orbiting planet. The immensity of the field alone makes this a difficult investigation. Even the exploration of the star closest to Earth, Proxima Centauri, is difficult to imagine. A round-trip voyage would take 8 years if the ship moved at a speed of 300,000 km per second and only photons can move at such speed. Even if the means of spacecraft propulsion were considerably improved, it would still take several centuries for a manned mission or even a probe to reach Proxima Centauri. Would there be any volunteers for such a long journey?

Any discovery of extraterrestrial life is unlikely to occur for many years outside the solar system. Despite this pessimistic outlook, progress can still be made in the field of astrobiology. The technical means currently at hand can indeed detect molecules in space comparable to those found in living matter or receive messages sent by faraway, intelligent extraterrestrial civilizations.

It has been known for several years that space is not absolutely empty. Thanks to spectrometers used in visible, ultraviolet or infrared light, and to radiotelescopes capable of detecting extremely weak radio waves emitted by molecules in the centimeter, millimeter and submillimeter range, hydrogen and helium atoms have been observed in space at very low concentrations (Figure 62). There are also other atoms in space as well as more complex molecules and a fine dust made of tiny grains of silicate and graphite, one tenth of a micrometer in diameter each. These grains originate from stars exploding at the end of their life. Hydrogen, oxygen, nitrogen and carbon atoms will stick to their surface. Having been brought together, these atoms will in time combine to produce water, ammonia and methane, all in a solid form. After tens of millions of years some molecules will break down into smaller elements or be transformed into free radicals. The hydroxyl radical ($OH^\bullet$) in particular is formed as water dissociates due to stellar UV radiation. After several million years the tiny grains might get close to a star. As the star heats the radicals and other molecules on the grains, they may recombine to form more complex molecules: water, methane and other molecules like hydrocyanic acid (HCN), formaldehyde (HCHO) and even ethyl alcohol (C_2H_5OH). Molecules containing up to 13 carbon atoms have been discovered. Currently, more than 60 such interstellar molecules have been detected, among which are organic molecules that can be found in living matter.

Interstellar molecules may provide insight into the speed at which the first stages of life or biogenesis could have evolved in the universe. Since these molecules may have played a role in the origins of life on Earth, their study has direct implications

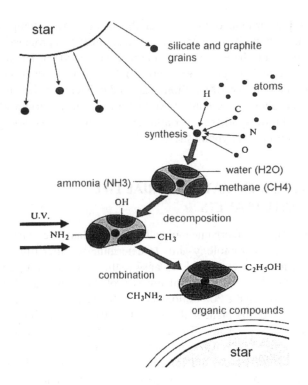

FIGURE 62 *Interstellar molecules and dust*

Space contains molecules (H-C-N-O) and tiny granules of silicate and graphite originating from stars that explode at the end of their life. After several steps and tens of millions of years, the radical OH, NH_3 (ammonia) and water recombine to form more complex molecules such as ethyl alcohol (C_2H_5OH), a compound present in wine.

in our understanding of terrestrial biogenesis. Space contains approximately one atom per cubic centimeter, which is obviously very little compared to Earth, where a cubic centimeter of gas (at a pressure of 760 mm of mercury and 0°C) contains 2.7×10^9 molecules. There are, however, cloud-like regions in space that are, 1,000 to 10,000 times denser. These clouds, essentially made of hydrogen, also contain more complex molecules attached to grains of interstellar dust. These regions being richer in organic molecules, they may foster the formation of more complex organic compounds and could even give rise to compounds such as plant cellulose.

The British astrophysicist Fred Hoyle believes that comets passing through these clouds would become charged with organic molecules. By associating with each other in the comet nuclei, these molecules might ultimately give rise to living matter molecules. Bacteria could develop and, if the comet hit the surface of a planet the climatic conditions of which were suitable, these bacteria could become the starting point of life. In that sense, life on Earth might be of extraterrestrial origin. If this hypothesis is correct, Hoyle suggests that laboratory experiments attempting to synthesize prebiotic compounds are bound to fail because they are based on the idea that life on Earth evolved from compounds formed in the primitive terrestrial atmosphere and then condensed in the sea or in lagoons. However, this failure may be temporary since our knowledge on the synthesis of compounds of living matter is progressing rapidly.

On the other hand, there is a more conservative view than Hoyle's which still accounts for the possible origin of extraterrestrial life. The Earth crosses interstellar clouds approximately every 100 million years and collects a billion tons of organic compounds. Such phenomena could have had a hand in the origin of life in conjunction with prebiotic synthesis on Earth itself. Numerous exobiologists, such as André Brack, support this hypothesis.

THE SEARCH FOR EXTRATERRESTRIAL LIFE AND HABITABLE PLANETS

The discovery of biological organic molecules in our galaxy is certainly fundamental but only a first step. Astrobiology aims to determine whether life other than ours exists and if the means are available to answer this anxiety- and passion-arousing question. Theoretically, extraterrestrial life is probable. Life can develop only on solid planets, and among the 200 billion stars of the galaxy, there may well be other solar systems with orbiting planets like ours. However, the question of whether such planets exist is still hotly debated. To date, over 80 exoplanets have been discovered. The first exoplanets were recently detected over a two-year period beyond the protoplanetary cluster near the star Beta Pectoris: two or three planets were found around pulsar PSR 1257+12, 1800 light years from Earth, and others around stars similar to the sun. They are large, about the size of Jupiter, and generally close to the star they orbit. The planet circling around 70 Vir, discovered by Geoffroy Marcy and Paul Butler from the University of California, is about 300 million light years away from Earth and might be habitable. However, discovering a planet is far simpler than showing that it is habitable. Life appeared on Earth under exceptional circumstances. If the sun were only 20% more massive than it is it would have used its fuel more rapidly and life would not have had time to develop. Moreover, because the Earth is 150 million kilometers from the sun, it occupies a narrow temperature zone where water can exist in the liquid state. Any closer and ocean water would have evaporated; a little farther away and the water would have remained frozen.

When the Earth was in its infancy, there was considerable volcanic activity. The volcanoes across the surface of the planet spewed water vapor, carbon dioxide and nitrogen. This phenomenon is called degasification. The water vapor precipitated as rain while the carbon dioxide spread throughout the atmosphere to form a barrier that trapped infrared radiation coming from the Earth. It acted like the glass of a hothouse and prevented the Earth from cooling down, thus providing an essential condition for the development of life. If the Earth had been larger and its radius a mere 10% greater than it is currently, there would have been more degasification, a greater greenhouse effect and the temperature would have been too high. Conversely, a smaller radius would not have been any more suitable. Computer simulations have shown that if the Earth's radius had been 6% less than it is, the atmosphere that would have formed would have been too thin to block UV radiation sufficiently. Only aquatic species protected by water would have therefore survived.

The presence of a large satellite like the moon also probably helped foster the appearance of terrestrial life. By playing a role together with the sun in the formation of tides, the moon helped create the alternate humidification and drying out of lagoons. Now, according to current theories on the origin of life, this is precisely where organic molecules might have concentrated and associated to form the first living creatures.

On the other hand, the Earth narrowly avoided a period of glaciation two billion years ago that would have led to complete freezing. In examining the highly specific conditions that led to the development of life on Earth, it becomes apparent that the mere existence of a planet does not make it habitable for all that. However, due to the vast number of stars in our galaxy and the likelihood that a good number are surrounded by planets, the possibility that some may support life comparable to or different from terrestrial life should remain under consideration.

THE SEARCH FOR INTELLIGENT EXTRATERRESTRIAL CIVILIZATIONS

If a planet suitable for the development of life were discovered, how would we detect the existence of living creatures? Because current technology does not allow direct observation, such extraterrestrial life could only be detected indirectly.

One way would be to identify compounds like methane, chlorophyll or oxygen on the planet. On Earth, oxygen originates from photosynthesis, a biological process that allows plants to absorb carbon dioxide, synthesize sugars and release oxygen in the process. Nothing like this has been found. Conversely, the presence of oxygen may not necessarily be indicative of life. The atmosphere of Ganymede, one of Jupiter's moons, contains oxygen as a result of the decomposition of water molecules, but this process is due to UV radiation and not photosynthesis.

A second way of obtaining evidence of extraterrestrial life would be to communicate with technologically advanced civilizations via radio waves. Although far-fetched, this method would certainly be conclusive. However, on Earth, of the 4 to 6 million species of living creatures—the exact number is unknown—only one so far has developed the capacity to communicate over such long distances. Given the odds, radio communication considerably limits the chances of success.

Indeed, a planet inhabited by bacteria, giraffes or chestnut trees would in all likelihood remain silent! In addition, if intelligent creatures inhabited a planet, they may not have reached an appropriate technological stage to be able to communicate across the galaxy. On Earth, life first appeared a billion years or less after the planet's formation 4.6 billion years ago. Multicellular species appeared only 600 million years ago (Figure 63). Man has existed for a mere 2.5 million years and radioelectric communication for less than a century.

Another possibility is that an extraterrestrial civilization might have reached an advanced level of knowledge and technology and then vanished, leaving undetectable life forms in its wake. As the French philosopher Paul Valéry pointed out, all civilizations are mortal. This mortality may be caused by nuclear war or natural catastrophes, particularly those originating from space. It is true that Man has been

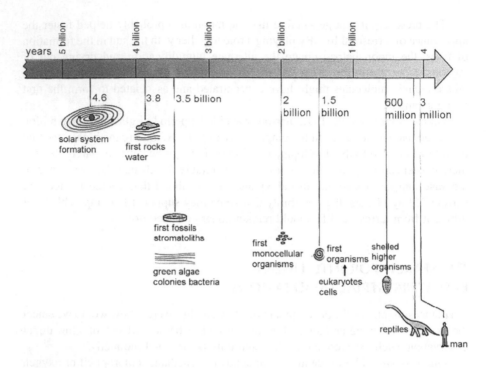

FIGURE 63 *Diagram showing the evolution of life on Earth*
The first living organisms appeared 3.5 billion years ago, perhaps earlier (3.8 billion years). The first steps of evolution were very slow, and the first nucleated cells emerged only 2 billion years ago. Multicellular organisms appeared 600 million years ago. Man has existed for a mere 2.5 million years and radioelectric communication for less than a century. If we extrapolate to other planets, the probability of discovering an intelligent extraterrestrial civilization appears to be very low.

responsible for the disappearance of some species due to technical advances, but tens of thousands of species have disappeared over the course of time, with a periodicity of about 25 million years. The Earth is certainly subject to major changes. For instance, the impact of a giant asteroid 65 million years ago resulted in intense volcanic activity and the disappearance of more than 70% of all species.

Additional factors may have also played a role in species extinction on Earth. For instance, the magnetic field, which acts as a shield against cosmic radiation, reverses itself every 100,000 to 1 million years. When this happens, the North Pole becomes the South and vice versa. A neutral magnetic state lasting for several million years would increase cosmic radiation and cause the partial destruction of the ozone layer that protects the Earth from UV radiation. This in turn could explain the disappearance of certain species. Finally, all terrestrial life is limited by the fact that the sun will one day transform itself into a giant red star that will burn the entire surface of the planet.

Fortunately, major cataclysms are very rare, and the sun will not burn itself out for another 5 billion years. Despite seemingly insurmountable odds, it is worthwhile to believe in the existence of intelligent extraterrestrial civilizations with which communication might one day be possible. The American astronomer Frank Drake has even attempted to define the possible number of such civilizations with the following equation:

$$N = N_g f_p n_e f_i f_i f_c f_d L$$

where N is the number of intelligent civilizations that have reached a stage of development allowing them to communicate by radio, N_g the number of stars in our galaxy, f_p the probability that a star is surrounded by planets, n_e the number of Earth-like planets in a planetary system, f_i the probability that the planet is inhabited, f_i the probability that an intelligent civilization can develop on the planet, f_c the probability that this intelligent civilization can find the necessary means to communicate, f_d the probability that it will wish to communicate and L the time (in years) during which this civilization will try to communicate.

This equation can obviously not be currently resolved. N_g itself remains unknown, although some estimate the number of stars in our galaxy to be close to 200 million. If, as James Kasting of the University of Pennsylvania argues, inhabited planets like the Earth must be at distances of 0.95 to 1.15 AU with respect to their sun (the AU unit being the Earth–sun distance, i.e., approximately 150 million km) and if 20% of all stars can have habitable planets, then only half the existing planets are situated in a so-called habitable zone. It is therefore possible that $n_e = 0.1$. Moreover, if binary and multiple star systems with unstable planetary orbits were discounted, only 10% of stars would be surrounded by planets and f_p would therefore have a value of 0.1.

Such a consideration would lead to a revised formulation of Drake's equation:

$$N = 4 \times 10^9 \ f_i f_i f_c f_L$$

Yet, even with this information, the equation is far from solved.

The possibility of communication does remain. In 1974, Cornell University sent a message using the 305-m-diameter radiotelescope in Arecibo (Figure 64). The message was sent toward the Hercules constellation, a region containing 300,000 stars. Unfortunately, it will take 25,000 years for the message to reach its destination, and another 25,000 years for an answer to return, assuming the extraterrestrial civilization responds immediately. To try and speed up this process, NASA and several European organizations created the SETI (Search for Extraterrestrial Intelligence) program. The aim of this program is to detect possible radio signals sent from faraway planets. As these signals are likely to be very weak, large radio telescopes and acute sensing devices are necessary to detect them. While Drake used a one-channel receiver, a 100,000-channel receiver was put in service in 1984, and receivers with several million channels are currently in use at different sites.[1] The sky is thus being observed at frequencies up to 25,000 MHz. A signal originating

---

[1] A channel corresponds to a determined frequency band for a given frequency range. Increasing the number of channels reduces the frequency band between each channel. The spectral resolution of the device is thereby increased.

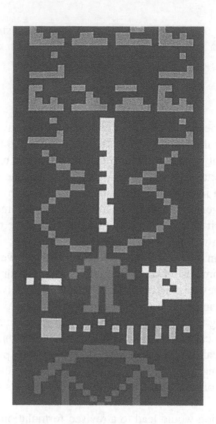

FIGURE 64 *The Arecibo radiotelescope message*

The message shows the DNA double helix, the atomic weights of hydrogen, carbon, nitrogen, oxygen and phosphorus, a human figure, the radiotelescope silhouette and the solar system.

from stars more than 1000 light years away can be detected. Of course, no signal has ever been detected to date, even after directing the monitors toward new planets. The chances of success are very slim, and it is for this reason that the American Congress abruptly decided to suspend all funding for this program in 1993. It was fortunately resumed with private funds, and SETI research continues with the collaboration of organizations such as the Planetary Society and the participation of many Internet surfers. In addition to radioastronomical studies, the detection of laser-pulse optical signals using optical telescopes is currently being pursued.

Conclusion

The search for extraterrestrial life is certainly one of mankind's greatest challenges. This quest is far from being resolved, even with the significant technological advances made in astronomy and radioastronomy. New research will be directed toward other planets in the solar system. Mars will receive particular attention, and we know that new automated missions will be carried out soon. In the near future, we may be faced with the issue of manned missions as well. The question is, should humans set foot on Mars? Certainly, but when?

The author remains optimistic since manned missions will probably always be justified. If the results from the Mars Surveyor-5 mission are negative, the argument could be made that an astronaut would have performed better than a robot. On the other hand, the discovery of Martian life would have such impact that a manned mission would be necessary. Exploring faraway hospitable planets directly has always been Man's dream. With this in mind, the words of the NASA administrator David S. Goldin should be applauded. During a World Space Conference held in Washington, D.C. in 1992, he said: "*If we consciously decide not to go to Mars, our generation will truly achieve a first in human history. We will be the first to draw a line and say to our children: this far, and no further.*"

Goldin's words may have indeed reached their audience. After the success of Pathfinder and thanks to Robert Zubrin's influence, NASA revived its Mars mission project. This project involves both cargo and manned missions with teams of six astronauts, all propelled by nuclear propulsion. A space station will be built on Mars, and astronauts will use vehicles to explore several hundred kilometers of the Martian surface. Humans are expected to walk on the planet between 2030 and 2050. A rocket capable of launching a 200-ton payload into low orbit and propelling 65 tons to Mars does not yet exist. The $40 billion or so necessary to accomplish this feat also remains to be found. It may therefore be too early to fix a precise calendar. It is obvious that the success of projects of this amplitude also depends on the economic situation of the United States and other contributing nations.

Epilogue

The issues that stem from the possibility that extraterrestrial life and intelligent civilizations exist are far from being resolved. The number of intelligent civilizations in the galaxy—defined as N in Drake's equation—is difficult to determine because of the number of unknown factors and the extreme variability of the factors we do understand.

Based on the immense number of stars in the galaxy and the presence of prebiotic compounds, an optimistic estimation of the number of intelligent civilizations could be on the order of several thousands. Moreover, living creatures are able to adapt to variable and often hostile environments. The appearance of life could occur as part of the evolutionary process of a planet.

Even if there is a high probability of extraterrestrial life, the chances that planetary evolution generated a species similar to ours are very slim. The human species is extraordinary because of its consciousness and psyche, both of which separate it from other animals. It is extraordinary as well for its capacity to think. For the first time, a being made of matter—elementary particles, protons, electrons and neutrons—is capable of contemplating matter. In a sense, matter is reflecting on itself, on its origins and nature.

Man is a species unlike any other because he spurns nature and will not stop until he has altered it. He also refuses his own nature in refusing death and has recently begun to resist genetic imperfections and even modify the course of natural evolution.

Should such an exceptional species, which consciously desires to bring itself closer to an omniscient and all-powerful God, be concerned that it is alone in the middle of the universe? Should we adopt the anthropical principle, which states that the universe is what it is so that life might develop to let a conscious being observe it? Other universes may have developed following the initial big bang, obeying different physical laws, different fundamental constants and offering no possibilities for biological evolution. How are cosmological evolution and human presence linked together? Some, like Sagan and Drake, believe that planetary biological evolution inevitably leads to civilizations like ours. Nothing, unfortunately, can prove or disprove this hypothesis.

Regardless of the incomplete knowledge about these issues where physics, biology and philosophy become intertwined, it is likely that Man will no longer be alone in the cosmos in the coming centuries, as he expands to colonize other planets.

When this day comes, biologists and physicians will have resolved the problems raised by the conquest of space. Let us hope that they will not forget the work of the pioneers who, under the sceptical and critical eye of their contemporaries, founded the basis of space biology and medicine.

References

Desplanches, D., Mayet, M.H., Ilyina-Kakueva, E.I., Sempore, B., and Flandrois, R. Skeletal muscle adaptation in rats flown on Cosmos 1667. *J. Appl. Physiol.* 1990, 68: 48–52.

Gasset, G., Tixador, R., Eche, B., Lapchine, L., Moatti, N., Toorop, P., and Woldringh, C. Growth and division of *Escherichia coli* under microgravity conditions. *Microbiology* 1994 (145): 111–120.

Hammond, T.G., Lewis, F.C., Goodwin, T.J., Linnehan, R.M., Wolf, D.A., Hire, K.P., Campbell, W.C., Benes, E., O'Reilly, K.C., Globus, R.K., and Kaysen, J.H. Gene expression in space. *Nat. Med.* 1999 (4): 359.

Horneck, G. Impact of microgravity on radiobiological processes and efficiency of DNA repair. *Mut. Res.* 1999 (430): 221–228.

Kacena, M.A., Merrell, G.A., Manfredi, B., Smith, E.E., Klaus, D., and Todd, P. Bacteria growth in space flight: logistic growth curve parameters for *Escherichia coli* and *Bacillus subtilis*. *Appl. Microbiol. Biotechnol.* 1999 (51): 229–234.

Moore, D., Bie, P., and Oser, H. *Biological and Medical Research in Space*. Springer, New York, 1996.

Nicogossian, A., Leache Huton, C., and Pool, S. *Space Physiology and Medicine*. Lea & Febiger, Philadelphia, 1994.

Perbal, G. and Driss Ecole, D. Sensitivity to gravistimulus of lentil seedling roots grown in space during the IML 1 mission of Spacelab. *Physiol. Plant* 1994 (90): 313–318.

Perbal, G., Driss Ecole, D., Rutin, J., and Salle, G. Graviperception of lentil seedling roots grown in space (Spacelab D1 mission). *Physiol. Plant* 1987 (70): 119–126.

Philpott, D.E., Corbett, R., Turnbill, C., Black, S., Dayhoff, D., McGourty, L.R., Harrision, G., and Savick, I.L. Retinal change in rats flown on Cosmos 936: a cosmic ray experiment. *Aviat. Space Environ. Med.* 1980 (51): 556–562.

Planel, H., Tixador, R., Nefedov, Yu., Gretchko, G., Richoilley, G., Bassler, R., and Monrozies, R. Space flight effects on *Paramecium tetraurelia* flown aboard Salyut 6 in the Cytos I and Cytos M experiments. *Adv. Space Res.* 1981 (1): 95–100.

Planel, H., Richoilley, G., Tixador, R., Templier, J., Bes, J.C., and Gasset, G. *The "Paramecium Experiment" Demonstration of a Role of Microgravity on Cell in Scientific Results of the German Spacelab Mission D1*. DFVLR Publishing, Ed. P.R. Sahm, D1, 1986, 376–381.

Planel, H., Soleilhavoup, J.P., Tixador, R., Richoilley, G., Conter, A., Croute, F., Caratero, C., and Gaubin, Y. Influence on cell proliferation of background radiation or exposure to very low, chronic γ radiation. *Health Physics* 1987 (52): 571–579.

Reitz, G. Radiation environment in the stratosphere. *Radiat. Protection Dosimetry* 1993 (1): 5–29.

Richoilley, G., Tixador, R., Gasset, G., Templier, J., and Planel, H. Preliminary results of the "Paramecium" experiment. *Naturwissenschaften* 1986 (73): 404–406.

Seibert, G. *World without Gravity* (research in space for health and industrial processes). European Space Agency SP 2001, 1251.

Tixador, R., Richoilley, G., Gasset, G., Templier, J., Bes, J.C., Moatti, N., and Lapchine, L. Study of minimal inhibitory concentration of antibiotics on bacteria cultivated in vitro in space (cytos 2 experiment). *Aviation, Space and Environ. Med.* 1985 (56): 748–751.

165

Vico, L., Chappard, Palles, S., Bakulin, A.V., and Alexandre, C. Trabecular bone remodeling after seven days of weightlessness exposure (Biocosmos, 1967). *Amer. J. Physiol.* 1988 (255): 243–247.

Vico, L., Lafage-Prouste, M.H., and Alexandre, C. Effects of gravitational changes on the bone system in vitro and in vivo. *Bone* 1998 (22): 958–1003.

Index

A

Absorbed dose, 128
Accelerations
  biological consequences of, 21
  effects on plants, 105
Accidents in space
  Apollo-13 mission, 13–14
  Challenger space shuttle, 14–17
  history of, 12–13
Acoustical detectors, on Huygens Cassini
    mission, 148
Actinomyces, 91
Adaptation to weightlessness, 45, 93
  by cardiovascular system, 46
  of vestibular system, 80–81
Adenosine triphosphate (ATP), fundamental role
    in living matter, 141
Adrenal cortex, 41
  hormonal regulation of collagen synthesis, 54
Aerobee-3 probe, 38
Aeronautical doctors, 22
Aging process, free radicals and ionizing radiation
    in, 126
Aldosterone, 41
  decrease in weightless state, 44
Aldrin, Edwin, 9
AlH84001 meteorite, 150
Alkaline phosphatase, role in bone formation, 51
Alpha particles
  causing greater damage than X-rays, 128
  in galactic cosmic rays, 123
Amino acids
  found in meteorites, 149
  prebiotic compounds necessary to synthesize, 146
Amphibian eggs, reproduction experiments in
    space, 113–116
Amyloplasts, response to gravity, 107–108, 110
Anatomic effects, of ionizing radiation, 126
Anderson, Michael P., 5
Anemia in space, 84–87, 92
Animal studies
  cardiovascular responses to weightlessness, 37
  early American, 37
  early Soviet tests, 39
  early space flights, 7–8

effects of gravity on skeletal system, 54–55
of muscle fiber changes in weightlessness,
    65–66
of skeletal changes in weightlessness, 57
of vestibular system adaptation in
    space, 80–81
spider vestibular system adaptation, 80–81
Anthropical principle, 163
Antidiuretic hormone (ADH), 41
Antigravity suits, 22
Antiorthostatic hypokinesia, 35, 61
Aorta, 40
Apollo program, 1, 9–10
  accidents in, 12–13
  purported UFO sightings during, 152–153
Apollo-1 mission, 12
Apollo-11 mission, 10
Apollo-13 mission, 13–14
Apollo-16 mission, heavy ion monitoring on, 134
Apollo-7 mission, 9
Arabidopsis
  increased mutation rates in space, 139
  microgravity experiments with, 109–110
Archimedes push, 118
Ares Vallis, 146
Argon, in atmosphere of Titan, 146
Ariane rocket, 2
Armstrong, Neil, 2, 9, 10
Around the World in 80 Days, 32
Arrhenius, S.A., 152
Artemia cysts, effects of space flight on, 137
Arterial pressure, in weightless state, 45
Arterial system, 39
Artria, 40
Aspergillus fungi, 24
Asteroids
  extraterrestrial life contained on, 149
  missions to, 17
Astrobiology, 141
Astronautics, 1, 18
  role of Tsiolkovsky in, 31–32
Atlantis shuttle, 17
Atlas rocket, 38
Atrial natriuretic peptide (ANP), 41
  sudden release in weightless state, 44
Auricular fibrillation, NASA solutions for, 95

167

B

B lymphocytes, 87
Back pain, associated with skeletal changes in
    microgravity, 55
Background radiation, 131
Bacterial life
    biogenesis of, 155
    fossils on meteorites, 150
    isolated on Venus, 149
    search on Mars, 142–143
Ballistic missiles, microgravity in, 34
Bed rest
    effect on bone mass, 54
    experiments in, 60
    muscular atrophy due to, 64
    simulating microgravity via, 35
Benton, E.V., 128
Beta Pectoris, 156
Bioastronomy, 141
BIOBLOC experiments, 135
Bioflight-1 probe, 38
Biogenesis, evidence from interstellar molecules,
    154–155
Biological experiments in space, 3
    cell division in weightlessness, 99–101
    cell membrane experiments, 101–102
    cellular energy metabolism in weightlessness,
        103
    cytoskeleton experiments, 102–103
    genetic effects of microgravity, 103–104
    Mars missions, 142–143
Biomedical Problem Institute, 61
Bion-10 biosatellite, 59
Biorak module, 17
    plant morphology experiments on, 110
Biosatellite Cosmos flights, heavy ion monitoring
    in, 134
Biosatellite-2, 38
    cell division experiments on, 99
    plant morphology experiments on, 108–109
Biosatellite-3, 38
Biostack experiments, 134, 135
Biosynthesis phenomena, 144
Biotechnology, new advances based on space
    flight research, 95
Bird legs effect, 43, 45
Birefringence studies, 103
Bleeding disorders, due to cosmic
    radiation, 131
Blood flow
    effects of space flights on, 92
    effects of weightlessness on, 83–87
    increased in weightless state, 46
    studying via suspended rat technique, 35–36

Blood perfusion, under conditions of weightless-
    ness, 91
Blood weight
    controlled by gravity, 41
    increased during accelerations, 21
Blue algae, effects of cosmic radiation on, 131
Body water content, decreased in microgravity, 45
Bondarenko, Valentina, 7
Bone development process, 49–53, 51
    and surface tension, 118–119
    effects of space flights on, 92
Bone fragility, due to exposure to weightlessness,
    49
Bone growth, microgravity effects on, 59
Bone loss
    after return to earth, 60
    hormonal regulation of, 56
    on disappearance of mechanical constraints, 54
Bone marrow, damage from ionizing radiation,
    127, 131
Bone resorption, 52
    effects of microgravity on, 57
    increased in microgravity, 56, 58
    stimulated by parathyroid hormone, 53
Booster mounting device, 15
Boosters, 15, 21
Brahe, Tycho, 122
Briegleb, Wolfgang, 35
Brown, David M., 5
Butler, Paul, 156

C

Calcitonin, 54
Calcium
    decreased on cellular level in space, 100
    dietary intake and bone mass retention in
        space, 60
    exchange between blood and bone, 53
    intestinal absorption of, 53
    physiological roles of, 49
    urinary excretion of, 54
Calcium homeostasis, 53
Calcium loss, in space, 49
Calcium metabolism, changes induced by
    microgravity, 55
Carbon dioxide, in atmosphere of Venus, 148
Carcinogenesis
    as delayed/late effect of radiation damage,
        138–140
    cosmic radiation and, 131
    heavy ion radiation and, 140
    ionizing radiation and, 127
Cardiac cavities, hypertrophy in microgravity, 44

Cardiac volume, changes in response to weight-lessness, 46
Cardiovascular deconditioning, 47
Cardiovascular experiments in space, 17
Cardiovascular system
    developmental abnormalities in space, 113
    effects of weightlessness on, 37
    physiology of, 39–41
    responses to microgravity, 45–48
Carotid artery, 40
Cassini spacecraft, 148
Cassini, Jean-Dominique, 147–148
Catabolism, increased in muscle fibers in microgravity, 66–67
Cataracts, induced by ionizing radiation, 127
Cell death, due to heavy ions, 133
Cell division, experiments in space, 99–101
Cell proliferation rate
    effects of microgravity on, 99
    increased in *paramecium*, 100
Cell-mediated immune response, 88
Cells
    effects of gravity on, 97–104
    effects of ionizing radiation on, 126
Cellular volume, increased in microgravity conditions, 100
Central nervous system (CNS), 40
Central venous pressure, changes in response to weightlessness, 46
Cerebral blood flow, increased in weightless state, 46
Chaffee, Roger, 12
Challenger D1 mission, 3
Challenger space shuttle, 14–17
    plant morphology experiments on, 110
Chawla, Kalpana, 5
Chemosynthesis phenomena, 144
Chlamydomonas, 100
Chretien, Jean-Loup, 24, 44
Chromosomal aberrations, due to heavy ion exposure, 135
Chryse Planitia, 142
Circadian rhythms, effect of space flights on, 91–92
Clark, Laurel, 5
Clinostats, 35–36
    in geotropism experiments, 105–106
    use in cellular experiments in space, 98–99
Cloud-like regions in space, 153
Cochlea, 70–71
Cognitive phenomena, importance to vestibular adaptation, 78–80
Cogoli, Augusto, 100
Collagen synthesis, regulation of, 54
Colonization of other planets, 163

Columbia shuttle, neurobiological experiments on, 78–79
Comets, evidence for life in, 150–152
Communication, possibility of intrastellar, 159
Comparative anatomy and physiology, vestibular system studies, 80–81
Competition in space, 7–11
Conrad, Charles, 3
Controlled ecological life support system (CELSS), 25
Convection phenomena, 98
Cooper, Gordon, 92
Cooperation in space, 11, 17
Cortisone, 57
Cosmic radiation, 21, 22, 23, 25
    and timing of space missions, 129–130
    as limiting factor in long missions, 140
    composition of, 121–124
    cumulative effects of, 130
    delayed/late effects of, 138–140
    discovery of, 121
    dosimetry of, 127–130
    effects combined with weightlessness, 137–138
    effects of ionizing radiation, 125–127
    general effects of, 131–132
    heavy cosmic ions, 133–137
    increased during magnetic field reversals, 158
    primary and secondary, 124–125
    solar flares and, 132–133
COSPAR space conference, 13
Costs, of space missions, 2
Countermeasures, 94
    to microgravity effects, 48
    to skeletal atrophy in weightlessness, 60–61
Covey, Richard, 4
Crick, Francis, 152
Cutaneous infections in space, 90
Cytos experiment, 99, 100, 101
Cytoskeleton, effects of microgravity on, 102–103

D

de Groot, R., 104
Decalcification, 59
    from wearing casts, 35
    of weight-bearing bones, 56
Degasification, 156
Demineralization, 55
    effects of weightlessness on, 92
Detached retina, novel treatments for, 95
Developmental biology
    amphibian egg experiments, 113–116
    evolution and gravity, 117–119
    mammal research in, 117
    sea urchin and fish egg experiments, 116–117

Diaphyses, 49
Discovery shuttle, 14, 17
Diuresis, 41
    excessive in initial exposure to weightless-
        ness, 44
    increased in microgravity, 44
Dizziness, under weightless conditions, 77–78
DNA, fundamental role in living matter, 141
DNA damage, by ionizing radiation, 126
DNA repair, effects of microgravity and cosmic
        radiation on, 137–138
DNA synthesis, inhibited by weightlessness, 89
Dobrovolsky, Georgi, 13
Dose-equivalent, 128
Dosimetry
    discrepancy between local and global, 139
    of ionizing radiation, 127–130
Drake, Frank, 159
Drosophila experiments, 22, 39, 119
    delayed/late effects of cosmic radiation, 138
    DNA repair in space conditions, 138
    increased mutation rates in space, 139
    reproduction in space, 113
Duprat, Anne-Marie, 116

                            E

Ear infections in space, 90
Echinocytes, 86
Electromagnetic radiation, 122, 125
Embryonic development
    arrested/abnormal with heavy ion
        exposure, 135
    in amphibians, 114–116
Endeavor shuttle, 4, 16
Endochondral bone, 51
Endocrine experiments in space, 17
Endocrine gland, heart as, 41
Endocytosis, 101–102
Endolymph, 70–71
Energy metabolism, effects of weightlessness
        on, 103
Environmental factors in space, 21, 22
    reentry, 24–25
    temperature related, 23
    vacuum, 23
Epiphyses, 49, 52, 57
    effect of growth hormone on, 54
Erythropoeitin, 84, 85, 86
Escape systems, 14
    missing on space shuttles, 16
Escherichia coli, effects of microgravity on, 99
European Space Agency, 1, 16, 98, vii
    Huygens probe built by, 148

Evolution
    cosmological, 163
    interaction with gravity, 117–119
    of life on earth, 156–158
Exobiology, 25, 141
    and extraterrestrial origin of life on earth, 156
Exoplanets, 156–157
Expiratory reserve volume, 90
Explorer-1, 1, 123
Extra-vehicular activities (EVAs). See also Space
        walks
    danger of cosmic radiation damage during, 129
    repair mission examples, 4–5
    Skylab-2 mission, 3
Extraterrestrial life
    beyond solar system, 152–156
    building blocks of, 141
    evidence from comets, 151–152
    evidence from interstellar molecules, 154–156
    evidence from meteorites, 149–151
    in solar system, 141–152
    on Jupiter, 149
    on Mars, 141–146
    on moon of Jupiter, 149
    on Saturn, 148
    on Titan, 146–148
    on Venus, 148
    search for, 25
    search for habitable planets, 156–157
    search for intelligent civilizations, 157–160
    unidentified flying objects and, 152–153
Extreme climate conditions
    on Mars, 146
    on Venus, 149
Eye movement frequency, 92

                            F

Facial congestion, 43
    as response to microgravity, 37
Fast twitch fibers, 65, 66
Fish eggs
    developmental abnormalities in space, 113
    developmental experiments in space, 116–117
Flight dynamics, 21–22
Fluid movement, in human body, 43
Fokker Space, 36
Forward fall, 78
Fractionated doses, 128
Franco-Soviet experiments, 100
Free radicals, 126
Free-fall, 28–31
French-American joint probe, 18
From the Earth to the Moon, 32

G

Gagarin, Yuri, 7–8
Galactic cosmic rays, 121, 122–123
Galileo, 27, 118
Gamma rays, 122, 125
Gas chromatographs
  on Huygens Cassini mission, 148
  use in Martian experiments, 144
Gaseous exchanges
  as metabolic process on Mars, 142
  Martian experiments in, 144
Gauer, Henry, 46
Gemini flights, 11, 12
Genes
  damage from cosmic radiation, 132, 138–140
  effects of microgravity on, 103–104
Geotropism, 36, 105–108
Glucocorticoids, regulation of bone formation by, 54
Glycolytic metabolism, of white muscle fibers,
  64–65
Gogoli, Augusto, 89
Goldin, David S., 161
Gravity, 21, 27
  and amphibian egg development, 113–116
  and evolution, 117–119
  animal experiments pertinent to, 54–55
  effects at cellular level, 97–104
  effects on aquatic species, 119
  effects on cardiovascular system, 40–41
  effects on long bones, 49
  effects on muscular system, 64–65
  effects on skeletal system, 54–55
  effects on utricle and saccule, 70–71
  effects on vestibular system, 75
  gravitropic response in plants, 105–108
  influence at cellular level, 34
  internal representation of, 79–80
  readaptation on reentry, 24
  response of plants to, 36
  variation with latitude, 28
Gray units, 127–128
Great Magellan cloud, 122
Greenhouse effect, on Venus, 148
Gregoriev, Y., 128
Grigoriev, Anatoly, 61, 90
Grissom, Virgil, 12, 38
Growth hormone, 54, 57
Guarapari, Brazil, 131

H

Habitable planets, search for, 156–157
Haise, Fred, 13
Halley, Edmund, 27–28

Hatton, Jason, 104
Haversian systems, 49–50, 52, 54
Head tilt, effect on vestibular system, 72–74
Headaches, from space motion sickness, 76
Heart, as endocrine gland, 41
Heart rate, modifications in weightless state, 45–46
Heavy cosmic ions, 123, 133–137, 139
  delayed/late effects of, 139–140
Heavy ion accelerators, 136
Helium
  detection in space, 154
  in atmosphere of Jupiter, 148
Helium nuclei, in galactic cosmic rays, 123
Hemoglobin, effects of weightlessness on, 83
Henry-Gauer reflex, 44
Hess, Victor, 121
Hills, Alan, 150
Hooke, Robert, 27–28
Hormesis, 131
Hormonal reactions
  effect on muscle fiber atrophy, 67
  to microgravity, 44
Hormones
  regulating calcium and bone tissue metabolism,
    56
  role in calcium homeostasis, 53
Howship's lacunae, 52
Hoyle, Fred, 155
Hubble space telescope, 2
  repair of, 4–5
Human physiology experimentation, 17
Human presence in space
  philosophical justifications for, 2
  technological justifications for, 3–5
Humoral immunity, 87–88
Husband, Rick D., 5
Huygens Cassini mission, 147–148
Huygens, Christiaan, 146, 147–148
Hydrocyanic acid, in atmosphere of Titan, 146
Hydrogen
  detection in space, 154
  in atmosphere of Jupiter, 148
Hypergravity effects, 100
Hypokinesia, effect on muscle fibers, 65–66
Hypotension, induced by gravity, 42
Hypovolemia, 44, 45

I

Il'yim, E.A., 35
Illusions, due to vestibular disturbances, 75
Immobilization
  effect on bone mass, 54
  muscular atrophy from, 64
  simulating microgravity via, 34

Immune response, effects of microgravity on, 87–90
Immunoglobulins, 88
  effect of space flights on, 88
Inebriation of space, 32
Infectious events
  due to cosmic radiation exposure, 131
  higher frequency in weightlessness, 90
Inferior vena cava, 40
Infrared radiation, 122
Inner ear, 70–71
Inspiratory reserve volume, 90
Institute of Aeronautic and Space Medicine, 135
Institute of Biomedical Problems, 7, 31, 90
  paramecium experiments, 100
Institute of Biomedical Problems (Moscow), vii
Insulin, 57
Intelligent extraterrestrial life
  and panspermia hypothesis, 152
  estimating number of intelligent civilizations, 163
  search for, 157–160
Interferon, 88
International Commission on Radiological Protection, 128, 132
International space conferences, 13
International space station (ISS), 17
International Space Station (ISS) program, 5, 6
Interstellar molecules, 154–156
Interstitial fluid
  infiltration after exposure to weightless state, 44
  redistribution in weightless state, 45
Intervertebral disks, changes due to microgravity, 55
Intestinal transit time, increased under conditions of weightlessness, 91
Ionizing radiation
  biological effects of, 121
  effects of, 125–127
  from heavy cosmic ions, 133
  increased with altitude, 121

J

Jahn, T.L., 34
Jaris, Gregory, 14
Jupiter, prebiotic compounds on, 148

K

Kasting, James, 159
Kennedy, John F., 9
Kepler, Johannes, 122

Kerala, India, 131
Kerwin, Joseph, 3
Kidneys
  hormonal regulation of, 41
  physiology of, 39–40
Klein, Harold, 142
Knight, T.A., 36
Komarox, Vladimir, 11, 12
Kondokova, Elena, 19
Korabl-3 rocket, 39
Korolev, Sergei, 11
Kosygin, Aleksei, 12
Kovalev, E.E., 128

L

Labeled release experiments, 143
Laika, 7, 39
Lander missions, 142
Lasers
  laser-pulse optical signals for extraterrestrial communication, 160
  use in ophthalmology, 95
Lazarev, Vasily, 16
Leach, Carol, 44
Lentil plantules, effects of microgravity on, 106–111
Leonov, Alexei, 9
Lethal effects, of heavy cosmic ions, 136–137
Leukemia, heavy ion damage and, 140
Life science missions, 16
  on ISS, 17
Light flashes, and heavy ion fluxes, 136
Linear acceleration, effect on otolithic apparatus, 73–74
Liquid oxygen hydrogen, development as fuel, 31
Locomotion system, 63
Long Duration Exposure Flight (LDEF) probe, 23
Long-term missions, 48
  challenges to muscle system, 67–68
  cosmic radiation as limiting factor in, 140
Longitudinal bone growth, effects of microgravity on, 59
Lovell, Jim, 13
Lowell, Percival, 141
Lower body negative pressure (LBNP), 47
Lucid, Shannon, 19
Luna-15 probe, 9
Luna-3 probe, 11
Lunar missions
  history of, 9–10
  radiation doses during, 130
  Soviet unmanned, 11
  to construct permanent manned bases, 17

Lunar module, on Apollo-13 mission, 13–14
Lymphocytes
    activation in space flights, 88–89
    effects of weightlessness on, 102
    energy metabolism in microgravity, 103

M

Mach 1, 21
Magnetic field reversals, 158
Magnetosphere, 123
    reduced protection during solar protonic events,
        133
Maintenance missions, 5
Makarov, Oleg, 16
Mammals in space, 39
    Laika, 7–8
    reproduction experiments, 117
Managed panspermia, 152
Manned missions, 1
    future of, 161
Manned space flights
    future of long-term, 18
    future possibilities for, 17–20
    history of American, 9–10
    history of Soviet, 7–9, 10–11
    to Mars, 94–95
Marcy, Geoffrey, 156
Marine archeobacteria, 149
Mariner probes, 142, 144
Mars
    atmospheric content of, 142
    possibility of extraterrestrial life on, 141–146
Mars Global Surveyor, 146
Mars missions, 17, 94, 95, 142
    cosmic radiation doses during, 130
Mars Observer, 145
Mars Pathfinder mission, 18, 145, 146, 161
Mars Surveyor-5, 146, 161
Mars-96 probe, 145
Marthy, Hans-Jürg, 116
Mass, relationship to weight and gravity, 28
Mass spectrometers
    in search for extraterrestrial life, 154
    on Huygens Cassini mission, 148
    use in Martian experiments, 144
Materials science missions, 17
McAuliffe, Christa, 14
McCool, William C., 5
McKey, Christopher, 146
McNair, Ronald, 14
Mechanical constraints, relationship to muscle
        fiber strength, 65
Medical advances, 95

Medications
    combined with physical exercise, 61
    for space motion sickness, 77
    minimizing muscle atrophy through, 68
Mental rotation, 78–79
Mercury flights, 12
Mesland, D.A.M., 98
Metabolic activity, search on Mars for, 142,
        143–144
Metaphyses, 49
Meteorites
    ALH84001, 150
    from Mars, 151
    originating from Mars, 146
    search for extraterrestrial life from, 149–151
Methane
    detection on Huygens Cassini mission, 148
    in atmosphere of Titan, 146–147
Methyl acetylene, in atmosphere of Titan, 146
Microbial agents, effect of weightlessness on, 90
Micrococcus radiodurans, discovery on Venus,
        149
Microgravity, 23. *See also* Weightlessness
    adaptability of biological systems to, 92
    countermeasures to, 48
    delayed/late effects of, 138
    effects at cellular level, 97–104
    effects on blood, 83–87
    effects on bone remodeling, 56
    effects on cardiovascular system, 37–48
    effects on cell membrane, 101–102
    effects on cell proliferation rate, 99
    effects on cytoskeleton, 102–103
    effects on DNA repair, 137–138
    effects on energy metabolism, 103
    effects on immune response, 87–90
    effects on muscle fibers, 65–67
    effects on plants, 108–111
    effects on respiratory system, 90–91
    effects on statocyte structure, 111
    effects on vestibular system, 74–77
    genetic effects of, 103–104
    in ballistic missile flights, 34
    nystagmus modified by, 78
    physiological stress of, 25
    preventing osteoporosis in, 61
    root disorientation under, 106–108
    simulating via random positioning
        machines, 36
    simulating via water immersion, 35
    simulation experiments, 33–34, 34–36, 36
    theoretical arguments for cellular effects of,
        97–99
Microorganisms, search on Mars, 142
Miles, Judith, 80–81

Mir station, 19
    muscle fiber research on, 65
    neurobiological experiments on, 78–79
    skeletal research aboard, 56
    vestibular studies carried out on, 75
Mitochondria, in red muscle fibers, 64
Molecular effects of ionizing radiation, 126
Monocytes, percentage increased in space, 86–87
Moon, role in biogenesis, 157
Morey-Holton, Emily, 35
Morphological abnormalities, due to heavy ion
    exposure, 135
Multiple-stage rockets, 31
Muscle contraction, 64
Muscle hypertrophy, 64
Muscle mass, changes during space missions, 63
Muscular atrophy, 92
    from wearing casts, 35
    progressive in weightless state, 45
    proposed mechanisms of, 66–67
    under conditions of weightlessness, 65–67
Muscular system
    effects of gravity on, 64–65
    effects of weightlessness on, 65–67
    muscle contraction, 64
    muscle fibers, 63
    proprioceptive functions of, 69
Mutation rates
    in *Bacillus subtilis* and Drosophila, 139
    increased in space, 22
Myocardium
    contractility in weightless state, 46
    structural alterations in response to
        microgravity, 48
Myofibrils, 41

                                        N

Nanobacteria, on meteorites, 150
NASA Ames Research Center, medical spinoffs
    from, 95
National Aeronautics and Space Administration
    (NASA), 11, vii
    Cassini spacecraft by, 148
    medical advances from, 95
Nausea, from space motion sickness, 76–77
Nephrons, 30–40
Neurolab missions, 17, 79
Neuromuscular spindles, 69–70
Neurospora, 91
Neutrinos, 125
Newton, Sir Issac, 28
Nicollier, Claude, 4
Nitrogen, in atmosphere of Titan, 146

Nitrogen losses, under conditions of weight-
    lessness, 67
Nonstochastic effects, of ionizing radiation, 127,
    131
Nystagmus, 77–78

                                        O

O-rings, 15
Oculovestibular interactions, 74–77
Oka, Mariko, 108
Oniwuka, Ellison, 14
Ophthalmology, medical advances from
    NASA, 95
Orbiter missions, 142
Organic compounds, degradation on Mars, 144
Orthostatic intolerance, 47, 48
Osteoblasts, 51
Osteoclasts, 51–52
Osteocytes, 50
Osteogenesis, 52
    reduced in animal studies during space
        flights, 57
Osteon lamellae, 50
Osteoporosis, 57
    delayed by heightened calcium intake, 60
    from exposure to weightlessness, 54
    preventing in microgravity, 61
Otolith apparatus, 74, 92
    disturbed under microgravity conditions, 71
    interaction with gravity, 72–73
    physiology of, 72
Otorhinolaryngology, medical advances from
    NASA, 95
Oxidative metabolism, of red muscle fibers, 64–65
Oxygen depletion, of blood in space, 84
Ozone layer, disappearance during magnetic field
    reversals, 158

                                        P

PAH family of hydrocarbons, 150
Panspermia, 152
Parabolic flights, 33, 34
Paradoxical sleep, 92
Paramecium experiments in space, 100, 103
    on effects of cosmic radiation, 131
Parathyroid hormone, 53–54, 54
Passive thermoluminescent detectors, 128
Penicillium fungi, 24
Perfusion pumps, 95
Photosynthesis, Martian organisms capable
    of, 143

Phylogeny, 117
Physical exercise
  benefits to muscle system, 67–68
  effect on muscle contraction, 64
  in prevention of space-related osteoporosis,
    60, 61
Physiology, advances made possible by manned
    space missions, 5
Pioneer probes, 148
  earth messages encoded on, 153
Planetary Society, 160
Plant cells, 106
Plant morphology, modifications in weightless-
    ness, 108–111
Plant orientation, effects of microgravity on, 105
Plasma volume
  decreased in response to weightless state, 47
  effects of weightlessness on, 83
  reduced in weightless state, 43
Polar regions, cosmic radiation doses at, 129
Poliakov, Valeri, 18, 78
Polynuclear leukocytes, 87
Postural phenomena, 78
  posture reflex modifications in rats, 117
  under conditions of weightlessness, 75–76
Prebiotic compounds, 163
  detection in search for extraterrestrial life,
    157
  from meteorites, 149–150
  on Jupiter and Saturn, 148
  on Titan, 146–147
Primary cosmic radiation, 124–125
*Principia Mathematica Philosophiae
    Naturalis*, 28
Promethazine, 77
Proprioception, 69–70
  illusions related to, 75
  vision compensating for, 92
Propulsion technology, 17
Protein kinase C, effects of microgravity
    on, 104
Protein synthesis, reduced under weightless
    conditions, 66–67
Proteus vulgaris, cell division experiments in
    space, 99
Protons, in galactic cosmic rays, 123
Protooncogenes, decreased cell division under
    microgravity, 104
Proxima Centauri, 154
Puffy face, 43, 44, 45
Pulmonary artery, 40
Pulmonary experiments in space, 17
Pulmonary vein, 40
Putsayev, Victor, 13
Pyrolysis release experiment, 142

Q

Quality factor, 128
Quantum gravitation, 28

R

Rad units, 127–128
Radiation belts, 121, 122, 123–124. *See also* Van
    Allen radiation belts
Radiation biology, 125–128
Radiation damage, estimating, 128
Radiation sickness, 127
Radioastronomical studies, 160
Radiotelemetry, 37
  in search for extraterrestrial life, 154, 157, 159
Ramon, Ilan, 5
Random positioning machine, 36
Rapid clinostats, 35–36
Readaptation, on reentry, 24
Red blood cells
  decreased production in space, 86
  effects of space flights on, 84–87
  rate of destruction in space, 85
Red muscle fibers, 64–65, 66
Red star, 158
Reentry, 24–25
  techniques to allow safe recovery during, 38
Rem units, 128
Renal stones, 60
Renin, 41
  reduced secretion in weightless state, 44
Repair missions, 5
Reproduction
  capabilities in space, 113–119
  genetic damage due to heavy ion impacts, 140
Residual volume, 90
Resnik, Judith, 14
Respiratory system, effects of weightlessness on,
    90–91
Reticulocytes, decreased under microgravity, 86
Retinal damage, due to heavy ion exposure, 136
Reusable space vehicles, v
RNA, fundamental role in living matter, 141
Rocket probes, simulating weightlessness with, 34
Rogers, William, 16
Root orientation, disordered under microgravity,
    106

S

Saccule, 70–71
Sagan, Carl, 148
Salamander egg experiments in space, 116

Saline solution, role in cardiovascular deconditioning, 48
Salyut missions, muscle fiber research on, 65
Salyut-7 orbital space station, 3
Satellite maps, 1
Satellite technology, 1
Satellites, uniform circular movement of, 30
Saturn
    life on moons of, 146–148
    prebiotic compounds on, 148
Saturn rocket, 153
Schiaparelli, Giovanni Virginio, 142
Schmitt, Didier, 104
Scobee, Francis, 14
Sea urchin eggs, developmental experiments in space, 116–117
Search for Extraterrestrial Intelligence (SETI) program, 159–160
Secondary cosmic radiation, 124–125
Semicircular canals, 70–71
Shepard, Alan, 38
Shoemaker-Levy comet, collision with Jupiter, 5
Short-sightedness, functional, 92
Shuttle flights
    muscle fiber research on, 65
    scientific programs aboard, 16–17
Siffre, Michel, 94
Single-cell organisms, studies of weightlessness in, 10, 38
Skeletal system
    animal experiments involving, 57–59
    bone development and restructuring in, 49–53
    countermeasures to preserve, 60–61k
    effects of space flights on, 55–57
    effects of weightlessness on, 37, 49
    influence of gravity on, 54–55
    relation to gravity and animal size, 118
    risks from space flight, 60–61
    role of hormones in, 53–54
Skeletal/striated muscle, 63
Skin burns, from ionizing radiation, 127
Skin infections in space, 90
Skylab-2 malfunction, 3
Skylab-3
    animal studies on, 66
    muscle fiber studies on, 65
Sleep-wake cycle, 91–92
    lengthened in space travel, 94
Slow twitch fibers, 65, 66
Smith, Michael, 14
Smooth muscle, 63
Sojourner probe, 146
Solar cycle, 129–130
Solar flares, 132–133
Solar Max satellite, 4

Solar protonic events (SPE), 132
Solar radiation, 23
Solar sail project, 152
Solar system
    search for life beyond, 152–156
    search for life within, 141–152
Solar wind, 121, 122, 124
South Atlantic anomaly (SAA), 124
    cosmic radiation doses at, 129
    light flashes and heavy ion fluxes over, 136
Soviet Academy of Sciences, 32
Soviet Biocosmos satellites, 135
Soviet biosatellite program, 35
Soviet Union, v
    history of early space flights, 7–9
Soyuz spacecraft, 6, 11
    reproduction experiments on, 113
Soyuz-1, 12
Soyuz-11, 13
Space anemia, 84–87, 93
Space biology, 25
    and early Soviet space flights, 7–9
Space cell biology
    cell division experiments, 9–101
    cell membrane experiments, 101–102
    cytoskeleton experiments, 102–103
    effects of weightlessness on genes, 103–104
    energy metabolism in weightlessness, 103
    theoretical arguments for effects of gravity on cells, 97–99
Space environment
    challenges of, 21–22
    flight-related factors and, 23–24
Space medicine, 5, 25, v
Space motion sickness (SMS), 76, 93
    temporary nature of, 77
Space rendezvous, Discovery shuttle and Mir orbital station, 17
Space Shuttle Columbia, 5–6
Space shuttles
    lack of escape systems on, 14
    neurobiological experiments on, 78–79
Space walks. See also Extra-vehicular activities (EVAs)
    cardiovascular adaptations to, 46
    history of early, 9
Spacecraft Progress, 6
Spacelab missions, 16
    Biorak module on, 17
    fruit fly reproduction experiments on, 113
    plant morphology experiments on, 110
Spontaneous fractures, 60
Spores
    inactivation by heavy ions, 135
    survival in space and extraterrestrial life, 152

Sputnik-1, 1, v
Sputnik-2, 39
  mammals aboard, 7–8
Spy satellites, 1
Star explosions, 122–123
Statocyte structure, effects of microgravity on, 111
Stochastic effects
  genetic damage, 132
  of ionizing radiation, 127
  risks for astronauts, 131–132
Streptococcus bacteria, survival in space, 24
Stress responses, to weightlessness, 27
Sulphuric acid, in atmosphere of Venus, 148
Superior vena cava, 40
Supernovae, 122–123
Surface temperature, of Titan, 147
Suspended rat technique, 35–36, 36, 58, 66–67
  and studies of microgravity effects on skeletal system, 55
Swingert, Jack, 13

T

T lymphocytes, 87
  decreased in space, 86–87
Tabony, James, 103
Tachycardia, as response to weightlessness, 45
Taylor, Albert, 142
Terrestrial attractive force, 28
Terrestrial magnetic field, 123
Testosterone, effect on bone matrix, 54
Thomson, D'Arcy, 119
Thornton, Kathy, 4
Thrust differential, 16
Tidal volume, 90
  decreased under conditions of weightlessness, 91
Timing, of space missions, 129
Titan, search for life on, 146–148
Tobacco plantules, increased mutation rates in space, 139
Totov, Gherman, 7
Transduction, 101–102
Tsiolkovsky, Konstantin, 31–32
Type 1 muscle fibers, 64–65
Type 2 muscle fibers, 64–65

U

Ubbels, G.A., 115
Ultraviolet radiation, 122, 151
  in early earth history, 156

Unidentified flying objects (UFOs), belief in, 152–153
Uniform circular movement, 30
Unmanned exploration, 1, v
Unmanned flights, 7–11, 18
Urinary calcium levels, increased in space flights, 56
Urinary infections in space, 90
Urination, increased in initial exposure to weightlessness, 44
Urodilatin, 48
Utopia Planitia, 142
Utricle, 70–71

V

V-2 rocket, 34
Vacuum conditions, 23
Valery, Paul, 157
Van Allen radiation belts, 2, 38, 123–124
Vasopressin, 41
  abrupt decrease in weightless state, 44
  use in space motion sickness, 77
Vasyoutine, Vladimir, 88
Venera probes, 148
Venous system, 39
Ventricles, 40
Venus, possibility of life on, 148
Verne, Jules, 31–33
Vestibular apparatus
  adaptation to space by, 24, 77–78
  comparative anatomy of, 80–81
  developmental abnormalities in space, 113
  effects of weightlessness on, 37, 74–77
  importance of cognitive phenomena to functioning of, 78–80
  plasticity of nerve centers, 77–78
  proprioception and, 69–70
  rat experiments in developmental biology of, 117
  vestibular system, 70–74
Vestibulo-ocular reflex (VOR), 74–77, 77–78, 78
Viking missions, 95, 142–143, 144
Vision
  improved acuity at great distances, 92
  undisturbed by weightlessness, 77–78
Visual acuity, effects of space travel on, 92
Visual system, developmental abnormalities in space, 113
Vital capacity, 90
  decreased under conditions of weightlessness, 91
Vitamin C, role in calcium homeostasis, 53
Vitamin D, role in calcium homeostasis, 53

Volcanic activity
  in infancy of earth, 156
  on moons of Jupiter, 149
Volemia in astronauts, 94
Volkov, Vladislav, 13
Von Braun, Werner, 34
Vostok-1, 8
Voyage to the Centre of the Earth, 32
Voyager probes, 146, 149
  messages encoded in, 153–154

W

Water, on Mars, 145
Water immersion, simulating microgravity via, 35
Water loss, in weightless state, 43, 44
Watson, James, 152
Weight, defined in physics, 28
Weight loss, in astronauts, 45
Weightlessness, 21, 23–24, 25, 27, v. *See also*
    Microgravity
  adaptation to, 45
  and amphibian egg development, 114–116
  and evolution, 117–119
  combined effects with cosmic radiation,
    137–138
  delayed/late effects of, 138–140
  described by Jules Verne, 32
  effects at cellular level, 97–104
  effects on blood system, 83–87
  effects on cardiovascular system, 37–48
  effects on cell membrane, 101–102
  effects on cellular proliferation, 100
  effects on convection phenomena at cellular
    level, 98
  effects on cytoskeleton, 102–103

  effects on energy metabolism, 103
  effects on immune response, 87–90
  effects on muscle fibers, 65–67
  effects on plants, 108–111
  effects on respiratory system, 90–91
  effects on skeletal system, 49–61, 55–57
  effects on vestibular system, 69, 74–77
  free-fall and, 28–31
  genetic effects of, 103–104
  hormonal reactions to, 44
  reproduced with rocket probes, 34
  root disorientation in, 106–108
  simulating on earth, 33–34
  simulating via bed rest, 35
  simulating via immobilization, 34–35
  simulating via suspended rat technique, 36
  theoretical effects at cellular level, 97–99
White muscle fibers, 64, 66
White, Edward, 3
World Space Conference, 161

X

X-rays, 122
Xenopus oocyte experiments, 115

Y

Young, John, 15

Z

Zond spacecraft, 11

Milton Keynes UK
Ingram Content Group UK Ltd.
UKHW040055071024
449327UK00019B/573

9 780367 454371